THE PEPTIDE PROTOCOLS BIBLE

3 IN 1

A Complete Guide to Enhancing Longevity, Vitality, and
Well-being | Targeted Strategies for Brain Boost,
Muscular Injury-Free and Body Optimization

Emerson Rowe

TABLE OF CONTENTS

INTRODUCTION

Peptides are short chains of amino acids that serve as vital signaling molecules in the body, influencing a myriad of biological processes. They operate on a cellular level to promote healing, regulate hormone levels, and enhance physical and cognitive performance. *"THE PEPTIDE PROTOCOLS BIBLE [3 IN 1]: A Complete Guide to Enhancing Longevity, Vitality, And Well-Being | Targeted Strategies For Brain Boost, Muscular Injury-Free And Body Optimization"* aims to demystify peptides, offering detailed insights into their functions and how they can be harnessed for therapeutic benefits.

The first segment, *"Peptide Essentials,"* lays the groundwork by introducing peptides and explaining their roles in the body. It delves into the science behind how peptides function and distinguishes them from proteins. The fundamentals of peptide therapy are covered, including synthesis, administration methods, absorption, metabolism, stability, and storage. Practical advice on starting peptide supplementation is provided, such as choosing the right peptides, determining dosages, timing treatments, understanding potential side effects, and adjusting protocols based on individual responses. This section also considers the ethical and legal aspects of peptide use.

The second segment of the book focuses on *"Peptide Protocols"* with targeted strategies for specific health outcomes. Detailed instructions on designing protocols for improved longevity, enhanced brain function, physical performance boosts, immune system strengthening, and hormonal balance optimization. Each protocol includes step-by-step guidelines for successful implementation along with advice on monitoring results to ensure maximum efficacy.

The final segment is dedicated to *"Peptide Health and Healing,"* illustrating how peptides contribute to healing processes in the body. There is thorough coverage of their anti-inflammatory properties, roles in tissue repair and regeneration, neuroprotective benefits, anti-aging effects, and improvements in metabolic health. It also addresses how peptides can aid in managing various diseases such as cancer, cardiovascular issues, autoimmune disorders, neurodegenerative diseases, and diabetes.

Furthermore, this book explores the role of peptides in mental health by enhancing cognitive function and reducing stress and anxiety while improving mood and sleep quality. It discusses their applications in reproductive health for both men and women including addressing menopause symptoms, supporting fertility, regulating hormones, and enhancing sexual health.

There is an enlightening discussion about cellular senescence—explaining how cells age—and how peptides can delay this process to sustain cellular efficiency. The immune system's interaction with growth hormone pathways is examined to highlight how it aids in cellular repair and overcoming pathogens.

Throughout this journey into peptide therapy, readers will receive practical advice for integrating these insights into daily practices aimed at long-term wellness. The book emphasizes ethical considerations while providing strategies for anti-aging lifestyles. With guidance drawn from trusted scientific literature and community support networks, this comprehensive guide ensures that anyone interested in peptide therapies will find valuable information tailored to their health needs.

BOOK 1
PEPTIDE ESSENTIALS

CHAPTER 1

INTRODUCTION
TO PEPTIDES

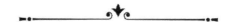

You might have heard about Peptides in a science class, seen them on the label of your favorite skincare product, or perhaps even encountered them when reading about fitness supplements. But what exactly are peptides, and why should you care? Peptides are short chains of amino acids. Amino acids, on the other hand, are the building blocks of proteins, which means that peptides are essentially mini-proteins. Think of them as little segments that combine in various ways to perform vital functions within our bodies.

There are 20 different amino acids that our bodies use to build proteins. When these amino acids link together in different combinations and lengths, they form peptides. If you imagine proteins as a train, then amino acids would be the individual train cars that make up that train. Peptides are like shorter trains or even just a couple of train cars linked together.

Now you might wonder why scientists and healthcare professionals pay so much attention to these tiny peptide chains. Well, it's because they play a surprisingly vast number of roles in our bodies. They act like messengers carrying signals from one part of the body to another. They're involved in several biological processes including healing, muscle development, hormone production, and immune system functions.

For example, insulin is one type of peptide hormone that regulates blood sugar levels. Without this peptide doing its job correctly, millions around the world would be unable to manage their blood glucose levels effectively – leading to conditions like diabetes.

Peptides can also help with healing and regeneration. Imagine you've got a cut or a bruise; specific peptides signal your skin cells to heal and regenerate faster. This naturally occurring process has been adapted into some skincare products designed to promote better skin health.

Another place where peptides have made a mark is in fitness and bodybuilding communities. Some athletes use synthetic peptides to enhance muscle growth and recovery times after intense training sessions. These synthetic versions mimic natural peptides to amplify desired effects such as increased muscle mass or faster recovery.

Not just confined to humans, but all living organisms rely on peptides for various functions like growth and immune responses. In plants, for example, certain peptides can act as defense mechanisms against pests or diseases.

In medical research too, scientists often focus on developing peptide-based therapies for conditions ranging from cancers to chronic pain because they can design these therapies to target specific cells without affecting healthy ones. It's almost like having a smart missile that hits only the bad guys while leaving the good ones untouched!

Peptides also display an interesting versatility; they can interact with many types of molecules within our bodies proteins, hormones, enzymes you name it! This makes them valuable in creating drugs and treatments tailored for precise effects while minimizing side effects.

By now you might see why understanding peptides matter—they practically run our biological show! From helping maintain optimal health through natural body processes (like regulating hormones) to promising advancements in medicine and skincare – these small chains pack quite a punch.

Classification and Types of Peptides

Understanding the classification and types of peptides is essential for several reasons. Firstly, Knowing the different types of peptides helps in understanding how they function and how they can be utilized therapeutically. Moreover, the classification can guide researchers and healthcare professionals in developing new treatments. For instance, antimicrobial peptides have gained attention for their potential to combat antibiotic-resistant bacteria. Without a clear understanding of peptide classifications, it would be challenging to develop such innovations effectively.

Classification of Peptides

Peptides can be classified based on several factors, mainly their length and functions. Let's break it down:

By Length:

1. **Oligopeptides:** These are short chains of amino acids, usually comprising 2 to 20 amino acids.
2. **Polypeptides:** These are longer chains that range from 21 to 50 amino acids.
3. **Proteins:** When the chain extends beyond 50 amino acids, it's typically considered a protein rather than a peptide.

By Function:

1. **Signal Peptides:** These helps direct the newly synthesized proteins to their appropriate destinations in the cell.
2. **Hormonal Peptides:** Examples include insulin, which helps regulate blood sugar levels.
3. Neuropeptides: These act as neurotransmitters in the brain, influencing things such as pain and emotions.
4. **Antimicrobial Peptides (AMPs):** Found in all living organisms, these peptides help defend against bacteria, viruses, fungi, and even cancer cells.

5. **Enzyme Inhibitors:** These peptides can inhibit the activity of specific enzymes; an example is ACE inhibitors used in treating high blood pressure.

Types of Peptides

Now let's zoom into specific types of peptides that you've probably come across or will find useful in various applications.

1. **Therapeutic Peptides**: These peptides are designed for medical treatments. They can target specific cells or tissues making them highly effective with fewer side effects than traditional drugs. Here are some common types:

   a. *Insulin:* Used for diabetes management.
   b. *Goserelin:* Used in cancer therapy and reproductive health.

2. **Cosmetic Peptides**: These peptides are widely used in skincare for their anti-aging properties.

   a. *Collagen Peptides:* Help promote skin elasticity.
   b. *Signal Peptides:* Trigger collagen production, reducing wrinkles and fine lines.

3. **Dietary Peptides**: Derived from food sources, these peptides can have health benefits when ingested.

   a. *Whey Protein Peptides:* Popular among athletes for muscle repair and growth.
   b. *Soy Peptides:* Known for their cardiovascular benefits.

How Peptides Work

To understand how Peptides work, think of them as messengers that deliver important information to various cells in our body, helping to regulate all sorts of biological activities. It's akin to sending emails within the body; they ensure that the right message gets to the right place at just the right time.

When peptides interact with cells, they bind to specific receptors on the cell surface. These receptors are specialized proteins that recognize and respond to certain signals. Think of these receptors as unique locks while the peptides are like keys. When the correct peptide (key) binds to its receptor (lock), it triggers a series of actions inside the cell. This can lead to a cascade of events within the cell, kicking off various biological processes.

Peptide-Receptor Interaction

One common way peptides work is through what's called signal transduction pathways. This might sound complicated, but it's essentially how cells process signals from outside and translate them into actions inside the cell. For example:

1. **Peptide binds to receptor:** The peptide attaches to the receptor on the cell's surface.
2. **Receptor activation:** The binding activates the receptor.
3. **Signal transmission:** The activated receptor sends a signal inside the cell.
4. **Cellular response:** The cell responds by doing things like turning genes on or off, producing new proteins, or changing its shape or movement.

A good example of how peptides work is insulin—a peptide hormone central in regulating blood sugar levels. When you eat, your blood sugar levels go up. In response, your pancreas releases insulin into your bloodstream:

1. **Binding:** Insulin binds to specific receptors on muscle and fat cells.
2. **Glucose uptake:** It triggers these cells to absorb glucose from the blood.
3. **Storage or use:** The glucose is either stored for later use or used immediately for energy.

OVERVIEW OF PEPTIDE FUNCTION	
PROCESS	**ROLE OF PEPTIDES**
Muscle Growth	Stimulate protein synthesis
Skin Health	Promote collagen production
Immune Response	Act as signaling molecules
Hormonal Balance	Regulate hormone levels
Weight Management	Affect appetite and fat metabolism

Aiding Communication & Coordination

Besides metabolic regulation akin to insulin's function, peptides coordinate other functions too:

1. **Muscle Growth & Repair:** Growth hormone-releasing peptides boost muscle growth by increasing protein synthesis.
2. **Skin Health:** Collagen peptides support skin elasticity and hydration by promoting collagen production.
3. **Immune System Modulation:** Some peptides act as signals in immune responses, alerting your body to invaders or injuries.

Therapeutic Uses

Given their pivotal roles, researchers create synthetic peptides for medical treatments—peptide-based drugs can manage a range of conditions like diabetes or even help in wound healing.

For example:

1. **Diabetes:** Lab-made insulin helps people who can't produce enough naturally.
2. **Pain Relief:** Certain peptides mimic endorphins (our body's natural painkillers).

Peptides simplify complex biological processes into manageable actions; understanding their roles can demystify many functions within our bodies and lead toward innovations in health and medicine.

Basic Science of Peptides

Just like Lego blocks can be combined in many ways to create different structures, amino acids combine in various sequences to form peptides, which can then perform a wide variety of functions. Amino acids are organic compounds that serve as the building blocks for proteins. They consist of an amino group (NH2), a carboxyl group (COOH), and a side chain unique to each amino acid. There are 20 standard amino acids that our bodies use to create proteins and peptides.

Peptides are defined by their length. Typically, a peptide is any molecule made up of 2 to 50 amino acids. If there are more than 50 amino acids in the chain, it is generally referred to as a protein. Peptides can be classified into various types based on the number of amino acids present: oligopeptides have 2-20 amino acids, polypeptides have 21-50 amino acids, and proteins have more than 50.

Peptide bonds hold these chains together. A peptide bond is a chemical bond formed between the carboxyl group of one amino acid and the amino group of another through a dehydration reaction (a reaction where water is removed). This bond forms a backbone for the peptide or protein chain.

The sequence in which the amino acids are arranged determines the properties and functions of the peptide. This sequence is known as its primary structure. Even small changes in this sequence can lead to significant differences in function.

Peptides serve many important roles in our bodies:

1. Some peptides act as hormones; insulin is one well-known example that regulates blood sugar levels.
2. Although enzymes are usually much larger proteins, some smaller enzymatic peptides exist that help in biochemical reactions.
3. Neuropeptides like endorphins act as signaling molecules between nerve cells.
4. Some peptides contribute to cell structure and integrity.
5. Certain peptides can function as antibiotics or play roles in immune responses against pathogens.

How do our bodies make these peptides? The process starts with DNA, which holds the code for each peptide. The relevant portion of DNA gets transcribed into messenger RNA (mRNA), which serves as a template for synthesizing peptides during translation processes inside ribosomes—the cell's protein-making machinery. There are also synthetic peptides—those created outside biological organisms—that mimic naturally occurring ones but can be designed for specialized applications, such as research or therapy.

One exciting application involves therapeutic peptides that target specific cells or tissues in the body. For instance, researchers are exploring peptides for targeted cancer treatments that could deliver drugs directly to cancer cells without affecting healthy tissues—potentially reducing side effects. In addition to medical uses, peptides show promise in skincare products due to their ability to penetrate the skin barrier effectively. Collagen peptides can promote skin elasticity and hydration, making them popular ingredients in anti-aging formulations.

The study of peptides extends across various fields like biochemistry, medicine, nutrition science, and even cosmetics. Some promising areas include new drug development aimed at chronic conditions like diabetes or auto-immune diseases. Understanding the basic science behind peptides opens up many potentials for future applications that could improve human health and wellness significantly. It's an exciting frontier that continues evolving with ongoing research and technological advancements. As we learn more about how peptides function at molecular levels, the possibilities seem almost endless—from treating diseases, and enhancing physical performance, to improving cognitive abilities and advancing skincare innovations.

Peptides vs. Proteins

Peptides are often involved in signaling within the body. For instance, insulin is a peptide hormone that regulates blood sugar levels. Another example is oxytocin, a peptide responsible for social bonding and reproduction.

On the other side, proteins are more diverse in their functions. Enzymes like amylase help digest carbohydrates while structural proteins like collagen provide strength and support tissues such as skin and bone. Hemoglobin, a protein in red blood cells, carries oxygen from the lungs to the rest of the body.

FEATURE	PEPTIDES	PROTEINS
Length	2 to 50 amino acids	50 or more amino acids
Structure	Simple chain	Complex 3D structure
Function	Hormones, enzymes, signals	Structural, functional
Examples	Oxytocin, Insulin	Hemoglobin, Collagen
Synthesis & Degradation	Quick	Longer processes

Synthesis and Degradation

The body synthesizes peptides quickly compared to proteins. This rapid synthesis allows peptides to act swiftly as messengers or regulators. Peptide degradation happens relatively fast due to their small size, enabling the body to quickly adjust their levels.

On the other hand, protein synthesis is a more time-consuming process involving transcription (copying genetic information from DNA) and translation (assembling amino acids into proteins). Because they form intricate structures, proteins are more stable but also take longer to break down.

Functional Roles

Peptide Functions:

1. **Hormones:** Many hormones like oxytocin and insulin are peptides that regulate bodily functions such as metabolism and reproductive processes.
2. **Neurotransmitters:** Certain peptides act as signaling molecules within the nervous system.
3. **Antimicrobial Agents:** Some peptides help in defending against pathogens by disrupting their cell membranes.

Protein Functions:

1. **Enzymatic Activity:** Enzymes are specialized proteins that catalyze biochemical reactions essential for life.
2. **Transport and Storage:** Proteins like hemoglobin transport molecules within organisms.
3. **Structural Support:** Collagen provides tensile strength to skin, bones, and other connective tissues.

Therapeutic Uses

Both peptides and proteins have significant therapeutic applications.

1. **Peptide Drugs:** Given their smaller size and ability to penetrate tissues easily, peptides make excellent drugs for targeting specific pathways without affecting whole systems. Examples include peptide-based cancer therapies and antidiabetic drugs like GLP-1 agonists.
2. **Protein Drugs:** Protein-based therapies have revolutionized medicine with treatments such as monoclonal antibodies for autoimmune diseases and cancers or enzyme replacement therapies for metabolic disorders.

CHAPTER 2

FUNDAMENTALS OF PEPTIDE THERAPY

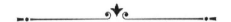

Because peptides can be designed to target specific cells or receptors, they offer a level of precision that minimizes side effects compared to traditional pharmaceuticals. For example, certain peptides can boost the immune system, improve wound healing, or enhance muscle growth, all while having minimal impact on other bodily functions.

Furthermore, peptide therapies are often derived from natural processes within the body, making them more biocompatible than synthetic drugs. This leads to potentially lower toxicity and better tolerance by patients. With advances in technology, producing synthetic peptides has become more cost-effective and scalable, making peptide therapy more accessible.

Due to these advantages, peptide therapies are being investigated for treating conditions like autoimmune diseases, cancer, diabetes, and even aging-related issues. The potential of peptides to address not just symptoms but underlying causes makes them a highly attractive option for modern medicine.

Peptide Synthesis

One important aspect of peptide therapy is peptide synthesis, which is the process of creating peptides in a laboratory setting. Understanding peptide synthesis can help professionals navigate this complex field more effectively.

Peptide synthesis involves linking amino acids in a specific sequence to form the desired peptide chain. This process can be done using either solid-phase peptide synthesis (SPPS) or liquid-phase peptide synthesis (LPPS), with SPPS being the more commonly used method due to its efficiency and ease of use.

Solid-Phase Peptide Synthesis (SPPS)

The SPPS method involves anchoring the first amino acid to a solid resin and then sequentially adding each subsequent amino acid. Various chemical reactions take place to ensure each amino acid bonds correctly to form the desired peptide chain. Once all the amino acids have been added, the completed peptide is cleaved from the resin and purified.

1. **Resin Selection:** In SPPS, choosing an appropriate resin is essential as it acts as the support for building the peptide chain. Common resins include polystyrene or Polyethylene glycol (PEG)-based materials.
2. **Amino Acid Activation:** Before they can be added to the growing peptide chain, amino acids must be activated to make them more reactive. This is typically achieved using agents such as carbodiimides or uronium salts.
3. **Coupling Reaction:** The activated amino acid reacts with the growing peptide chain anchored on the resin, forming a new bond.
4. **Cleavage and Deprotection:** After completing the peptide sequence, it must be cleaved from the resin and deprotected (removing protecting groups that shield reactive parts during synthesis).

Liquid-Phase Peptide Synthesis (LPPS)

Although less common than SPPS, LPPS is another method used for peptide synthesis. In LPPS, peptides are synthesized in solution rather than on a solid support. This approach offers some flexibility but is generally more time-consuming and labor-intensive compared to SPPS.

1. **Solution Preparation:** Like SPPS but taking place in solution.
2. **Sequential Addition of Amino Acids:** Sequential addition occurs similarly but requires careful manipulation since everything happens in a liquid medium.
3. **Purification Steps:** These steps are necessary multiple times throughout LPPS due to possible side reactions occurring more easily without a resin's stabilization.

Handling Side Reactions

One significant challenge in both SPPS and LPPS is minimizing side reactions that can lead to impurities within the synthesized peptides. These can include:

1. **Racemization:** The incorrect configuration of chiral centers.
2. **Deprotection Failures:** Failure to remove protective groups can impede final product purity.

Using highly purified reagents and optimizing reaction conditions helps mitigate these issues.

Purification Techniques

Once peptides are synthesized, purification becomes vital to ensure they are free from byproducts or incomplete sequences:

1. Chromatography Methods, especially High-Performance Liquid Chromatography (HPLC), are predominantly used due to their precision in separating different components based on their size or charge.

2. Lyophilization, also known as freeze-drying, helps stabilize the finalized pure peptides for long-term storage without degradation. This method removes water from the peptides after freezing, which aids in maintaining their structure and activity over time.

Validation of Peptide Purity and Integrity

Ensuring that synthesized peptides meet the required purity and functionality is crucial. Various analytical techniques are employed for this purpose:

1. **Mass Spectrometry (MS):** This technique helps verify the molecular weight of the peptide, ensuring it matches the expected value.
2. **Amino Acid Analysis:** This method confirms that the peptide composition aligns with the intended sequence.
3. **Electrophoresis:** Gel electrophoresis can be used to assess purity by observing the presence of any contaminating proteins or peptides.

Routes of Administration

Understanding the various routes of administration for peptide therapy is crucial for optimizing treatment efficacy and patient compliance. Each method offers unique benefits and drawbacks, and the choice of route will depend on the specific peptide being used, the condition being treated, and patient preferences. Healthcare providers must thoroughly evaluate these factors to determine the most appropriate administration route for achieving optimal therapeutic outcomes.

1. **Oral Administration**: Oral administration is the most common and convenient route for taking medications, including peptides. However, it is not always effective for peptides due to the harsh environment of the gastrointestinal tract. Peptides can be broken down by stomach acid and digestive enzymes before they reach the bloodstream.

Advantages: Convenient; Non-invasive; Easy to administer without medical assistance

Disadvantages: Low bioavailability; Risk of peptide degradation in the stomach

2. **Subcutaneous Injection**: Subcutaneous (Sub-Q) injection involves injecting peptides into the fatty tissue just beneath the skin. This method allows for slower, more controlled absorption compared to other types of injections.

Advantages: Higher bioavailability compared to oral administration; Relatively painless; Suitable for self-administration

Disadvantages: Requires knowledge of injection techniques; Risk of infection at injection site

3. **Intramuscular Injection**: Intramuscular (IM) injection delivers peptides directly into muscle tissue. This method allows for faster absorption than subcutaneous injections but can be more painful.

Advantages: Faster absorption than subcutaneous; High bioavailability

Disadvantages: More painful than subcutaneous injections; Requires precision and training to avoid damaging nerves or blood vessels

4. **Intravenous Administration**: Intravenous (IV) administration involves directly injecting peptides into a vein. This ensures that the maximum amount of peptide enters the bloodstream quickly.

Advantages: Immediate effect; 100% bioavailability

Disadvantages: Invasive; Requires medical professional for administration; Risk of infection or complications at injection site

5. **Transdermal Patches/Creams**: Transdermal methods involve applying patches or creams that enable peptides to penetrate through the skin and into the bloodstream.

Advantages: Non-invasive; Sustained release over time; Easy application

Disadvantages: Variable absorption rates depending on skin condition; Not suitable for all types of peptides

6. **Nasal Spray**: Nasal sprays deliver peptides through the nasal mucosa directly into systemic circulation.

Advantages: Quick absorption; Non-invasive; Easy to use

Disadvantages: Potential irritation of nasal passages; Variable absorption efficiency

7. **Sublingual Administration**: Sublingual administration involves placing a peptide under the tongue where it gets absorbed through the tissues lining the mouth.

Advantages: Quick absorption; Avoids degradation by stomach acids; Easy to administer

Disadvantages: Not suitable for all types of peptides; Limited volume that can be administered at once

ROUTE	BIOAVAILABILITY	SPEED	CONVENIENCE	INVASIVENESS
Oral	Low	Slow	High	Non-invasive
Subcutaneous	Medium	Medium	Medium	Minimally invasive
Intramuscular	High	Fast	Low	Low
Intravenous	Very High	Immediate	Low	Highly invasive
Transdermal	Variable	Slow	High	Non-invasive
Nasal	Variable	Fast	High	Non-invasive
Sublingual	Medium	Fast	High	Non-invasive

Absorption and Metabolism

When peptides are given, they start by being absorbed. Absorption is the process by which peptides enter the bloodstream from the site of administration. The efficiency and method of absorption can vary based on several factors:

1. **Molecular Size:** Smaller peptides are generally absorbed more readily than larger ones. Their smaller size allows them to pass through cellular membranes more easily.
2. **Stability:** Peptides can be susceptible to degradation by enzymes in the digestive system. Some peptides are chemically modified to enhance their stability and absorption.

3. **Transport Mechanisms:** Specialized transport proteins can facilitate the movement of peptides across cellular membranes.

Mechanisms of Absorption

Peptides can be absorbed through several mechanisms, primarily depending on their size and chemical properties:

1. **Passive Diffusion:** Small, non-polar peptides can diffuse passively across cell membranes along a concentration gradient. This means they move from an area of higher concentration to one of lower concentration without the need for energy.
2. **Facilitated Diffusion:** Larger or more polar peptides may require help from specific transport proteins embedded in cell membranes. These proteins assist in moving the peptides across the membrane without expending energy.
3. **Active Transport:** This mechanism requires energy (usually in the form of ATP) to move peptides against a concentration gradient. Active transport is essential for absorbing larger peptide molecules that cannot pass through cell membranes otherwise.
4. **Endocytosis:** In this process, cells engulf peptide molecules using their cell membrane, forming a vesicle that contains the peptide inside the cell.

Factors Affecting Peptide Absorption

Several factors influence how effectively peptides are absorbed into the bloodstream:

1. **pH Levels:** The acidity or alkalinity of the environment at the absorption site plays a crucial role. Certain peptides may degrade in highly acidic or alkaline conditions.
2. **Presence of Enzymes:** Enzymes, particularly proteases, can break down peptide bonds, affecting their availability for absorption. Inhibitors may be used to protect peptides from enzymatic degradation.
3. **Dietary Components:** Food intake can impact peptide absorption, with some foods enhancing or inhibiting their uptake.

Metabolism of Peptides

Once absorbed into the bloodstream, peptides undergo metabolism—a series of chemical reactions that transform them into active forms or breakdown products for excretion.

Stages of Peptide Metabolism:

1. **Enzymatic Degradation:** Peptidases and proteases are enzymes that break down peptides into their constituent amino acids or smaller peptide fragments. This degradation occurs primarily in the liver but also in other tissues such as kidneys and blood plasma.

2. **Modification Reactions:** Some peptides undergo modifications like phosphorylation (addition of phosphate groups) or glycosylation (attachment of sugar molecules), which affect their activity and lifespan. These modifications often serve regulatory functions, modulating how long a peptide remains active in circulation.

3. **Excretion:** Once metabolized, inactive fragments or waste products are removed from the body via urine or feces. The kidneys play a crucial role in filtering out these breakdown products.

The balance between synthesis, absorption, and metabolism determines the overall therapeutic efficacy of peptide treatments.

Peptide Stability and Storage

Peptide therapy offer treatments for a variety of conditions by harnessing the potential of peptides, which are short chains of amino acids. For those using peptide therapy, understanding peptide stability and storage is crucial to ensure the effectiveness and safety of the treatment.

Peptide Stability

1. **Sensitivity to Degradation**: Peptides are susceptible to degradation, which can render them ineffective. Factors that affect peptide stability include temperature, pH, and exposure to light and moisture. Peptides can degrade through hydrolysis (breakdown by water), oxidation (reaction with oxygen), and enzymatic breakdown.

2. **Temperature Sensitivity**: Peptides are often sensitive to temperature fluctuations. Most peptides need to be stored at low temperatures, with many requiring refrigeration (2-8°C) or even freezing (-20°C) for long-term storage. High temperatures can accelerate degradation processes.

3. **pH Levels**: Each peptide has an optimal pH range for stability. Extreme pH levels can lead to the breakdown of peptide bonds or cause aggregation, where peptides stick together forming unusable clumps. Maintaining the pH within the specified range as per the manufacturer's instructions is essential for stability.

4. **Light Exposure**: Exposure to light, particularly UV light, can lead to peptide degradation through photochemical reactions. It is advisable to store peptides in amber vials or other opaque containers that block light.

5. **Moisture Control**: Moisture can significantly impact peptide stability, especially for lyophilized (freeze-dried) peptides that can absorb water from humid environments. Storing peptides in a dry place and using desiccants can help maintain their stability.

Peptide Storage

Proper storage is essential to maintain the quality and effectiveness of peptides

1. **Refrigeration vs Freezing**

   a. *Refrigeration (2-8°C):* Suitable for short-term storage usually up to a few weeks. For several peptides, refrigeration maintains their potency without harming their structure.
   b. *Freezing (-20°C):* Recommended for long-term storage extending beyond a few months. Freezing slows down all processes that cause deterioration. However, repeated freeze-thaw cycles should be avoided as they can damage the peptide's structure.

2. **Lyophilized vs Reconstituted Form**

   a. *Lyophilized Powder:* Peptides are often sold in lyophilized form to enhance shelf life and stability at various temperatures. It's usually stable at room temperature until reconstitution.

b. *Reconstituted Solutions:* Once mixed with a solvent (usually sterile water or saline), peptides must be stored according to specific guidelines often requiring refrigeration or immediate use within days or weeks depending on the specific peptide's properties.

3. **Container Selection** Using appropriate containers is vital:

a. *Glass Vials:* Often preferred due to their impermeability and inert nature.
b. *Plastic Vials:* Should be chosen carefully as some plastics may interact with peptides or allow slight gas permeability.

GENERAL GUIDELINES FOR PEPTIDE STORAGE		
CONDITION	LYOPHILIZED PEPTIDES	RECONSTITUTED PEPTIDES
Room Temperature	Stable up to weeks	Not recommended
Refrigeration (2-8°C)	Stable up to years*	1-4 weeks
Freezing (-20°C)	Stable long-term*	| Few months

* *Subjected to individual peptide guidelines provided by manufacturers.*

4. **Avoiding Contamination**: Ensuring that reconstituted peptides remain uncontaminated is essential. Use sterile techniques when mixing peptides with solvents. Always utilize clean, sterile syringes and vials to prevent introducing bacteria or other particles.

5. **Avoiding Repeated Thawing and Refreezing**: Repeated cycles of thawing and refreezing can cause peptide degradation. To avoid this, it's best to aliquot peptides into smaller, single-use portions before freezing. This way, each aliquot can be thawed individually as needed, without affecting the rest.

Starting with Peptides

Peptide therapy involves using specific peptides to achieve desired health outcomes. These can include improved muscle mass, enhanced recovery, anti-aging effects, and better cognitive function.

1. **Targeted Action:** Unlike many broad-spectrum treatments, peptides work by targeting specific cellular functions.
2. **Fewer Side Effects:** Because they mimic natural bodily processes, peptides generally have fewer side effects compared to traditional medications.
3. **Versatility:** Peptides can be used to treat a wide range of conditions—from skin issues to metabolic diseases.

How to Start with Peptide Therapy

1. **Consult a Healthcare Provider:** Your first step should be consulting a qualified healthcare provider. They can help you determine which peptides may benefit you the most and at what dosages.

2. **Laboratory Testing**: Before starting peptide therapy, it's often advisable to undergo laboratory tests. These tests can provide a baseline for various biomarkers that peptides aim to influence. For example, checking your IGF-1 levels before starting a growth hormone-releasing peptide can guide dosage and expectations.

3. **Choosing the Right Peptides**

For General Wellness:

    a. *BPC-157:* Known for its healing properties and ability to enhance tissue repair.
    b. *Thymosin Alpha-1:* Boosts the immune system and may help fight infections.

For Athletic Performance:

    a. *CJC-1295/Ipamorelin:* Aids in growth hormone release for increased muscle mass and recovery.
    b. *TB-500:* Promotes healing and reduces inflammation.

For Anti-Aging:

    a. *GHK-Cu:* Improves skin health by promoting collagen production.
    b. *Epithalon:* Enhances telomere length, contributing to anti-aging effects at the cellular level.

4. **Sourcing Quality Peptides**: Make sure you're sourcing your peptides from reputable pharmacies or compounding labs. Ensure they follow good manufacturing practices (GMP).

5. **Administration Methods**: Most peptides are administered via subcutaneous injections, which involve injecting the peptide under the skin using a small needle. While this might seem daunting initially, most people get comfortable with it quickly. Other methods include topical creams and oral supplements, although these might have varying efficacy levels.

Injection Tips:

    a. *Clean the Area:* Always sterilize the injection site with an alcohol swab before administering the peptide.
    b. *Rotate Injection Sites:* To avoid local irritation or scar tissue buildup, rotate your injection sites.
    c. *Proper Storage:* Keep your peptides in a refrigerator to maintain their stability. Some may need freezing depending on their chemical structure.

6. **Monitoring Progress**: Track your progress through regular check-ups and laboratory tests. Keeping a journal where you note any changes—positive or negative—can also be beneficial for adjusting dosages or switching peptides if necessary.

While peptide therapy is generally safe, it's essential to be aware of potential side effects like:

- ☐ Localized irritation at injection sites
- ☐ Allergic reactions
- ☐ Hormonal imbalances if taken excessively

Should you experience any severe reactions, consult your healthcare provider immediately.

CHAPTER 3

PEPTIDE SUPPLEMENTATION BASICS

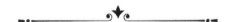

Peptide supplementation can help address specific needs that ordinary nutrients might not cover. Peptides are short chains of amino acids that act as building blocks for proteins essential to myriad bodily functions, including muscle repair, hormone regulation, and immune function. By supplementing your diet with peptides, you can support these critical processes more effectively.

Furthermore, supplementation allows for targeted health benefits. You can select specific peptides that match your health goals—whether that's improved athletic performance, better skin health, or enhanced cognitive function. This selectivity makes peptide supplementation an efficient way to enhance overall well-being.

Choosing the Right Peptides

The first step in selecting the right peptide supplementation is identifying your goals. Are you looking to enhance muscle recovery, boost cognitive function, improve skin health, or support weight loss? Different peptides serve different purposes, so knowing what you want to achieve will help narrow down your options.

1. **BPC-157:** Known for its healing properties, BPC-157 is commonly used to accelerate recovery from injuries and reduce inflammation. Athletes and those recovering from surgery might find this peptide particularly useful.
2. **CJC-1295 with DAC (Drug Affinity Complex):** This is a growth hormone-releasing hormone (GHRH) analogue that helps increase growth hormone levels. It's often used for anti-aging purposes and to improve physical performance by promoting muscle growth and fat loss.

3. **GHRP-6:** Growth Hormone Releasing Peptide-6 stimulates the release of growth hormone (GH). Besides its use in muscle growth and weight loss, it also enhances recovery and supports overall vitality.

4. **Thymosin Beta-4 (TB-500):** This peptide is celebrated for its ability to promote wound repair and muscle recovery. It is especially beneficial for people dealing with soft tissue damage or wishing to speed up post-exercise recovery.

5. **Melanotan II:** Popular among those seeking a tan without sun exposure, Melanotan II stimulates the production of melanin. It also has appetite-suppressing properties that might aid in weight management.

6. **Epithalon:** This peptide has been linked to anti-aging benefits by promoting better sleep, enhancing mood, and supporting overall longevity.

Dosage Guidelines

When starting peptide supplementation, determining the appropriate dosage is crucial. Each peptide has specific dosage recommendations based on its intended benefits and the individual's physiological makeup. Here's a breakdown of common peptides and their typical dosages:

PEPTIDE	DOSAGE RANGE	NOTES
BPC-157	200-800 mcg per day	Ideal for injury recovery and reducing inflammation
CJC-1295 with DAC	2 mg per week	Enhances muscle growth and fat loss; long-lasting effects
GHRP-6	100-300 mcg 2-3 times per day	Stimulates growth hormone release; good for muscle gain and fat loss
Thymosin Beta-4 (TB-500)	2-10 mg per week	Accelerates healing processes and reduces inflammation
Melanotan II	Initial: 250 mcg daily; Maintenance: 500-1000 mcg per week	Induces tanning; can reduce appetite as a side effect
Epithalon	5-10 mg per day for 10-20 days	Anti-aging benefits; improves sleep and immune system

Timing and Frequency

Just as important as dosage is the timing and frequency of peptide supplementation. Each peptide works differently, and its effects can be optimized by administering it at specific times.

1. **BPC-157:** Administer BPC-157 daily. This peptide is usually injected subcutaneously (under the skin) or intramuscularly (directly into muscles). Depending on the severity of the injury or inflammation, your dosage may be divided into two smaller doses taken morning and evening.

2. **CJC-1295 with DAC:** Taken once weekly, due to its long half-life. A single injection of 2 mg per week is sufficient to reap its benefits. This peptide is best administered in the evening before bedtime to align with the body's natural growth hormone release cycle.

3. **GHRP-6:** GHRP-6 should be taken two to three times daily, particularly before meals due to its impact on hunger. Injecting 100 to 300 mcg each time provides optimal results. It's advisable not to eat within an hour after injection to enhance the peptide's efficacy.

4. **Thymosin Beta-4 (TB-500):** Dosages range from 2 mg up to 10 mg weekly based on individual needs. For initial treatments aimed at rapid healing, higher doses may be administered split into two weekly injections. Maintenance doses are generally lower.

5. **Melanotan II:** Start with a small dose of 250 mcg daily to assess tolerance for about a week before moving on to maintenance dosages. Once tolerance is established, it can be administered at 500 mcg to 1000 mcg weekly. This peptide is typically injected subcutaneously.

6. **Epithalon:** For anti-aging purposes, Epithalon is taken in short-term cycles ranging from ten to twenty days straight. The daily dosage lies between 5 mg and 10 mg, generally split into two doses taken morning and evening.

While determining dosage and timing might seem intricate, these guidelines help create an effective regimen tailored to individual needs. Always consulting with a healthcare professional before starting any supplementation can ensure safety and efficacy.

Potential Side Effects

When using peptides, it's important to be aware of potential side effects. Possible adverse reactions can differ based on the specific peptide being used.

Common Side Effects

1. **BPC-157:** Usually, well-tolerated but may cause dizziness or digestive upset.
2. **CJC-1295 with DAC:** Possible adverse effects include fatigue, headaches, and fluid retention.
3. **GHRP-6:** Common side effects are increased hunger, water retention, and temporary pain at the injection site.
4. **Thymosin Beta-4 (TB-500):** Generally mild side effects but may include redness at the injection site.
5. **Melanotan II:** Often causes nausea and flushing; may also increase libido.
6. **Epithalon:** Generally, very few side effects but reports include potential digestive disturbances.

Monitoring these side effects is an essential part of peptide therapy to ensure safe and effective use.

Monitoring and Adjusting Treatment

Proper monitoring is key to achieving optimal results from peptide supplementation. Here's how you can keep track:

1. **Initial Baseline Testing:** Before starting any new peptide regimen, it's advisable to get baseline blood tests. This might include hormone levels (if using GHRP-6 or CJC-1295 with DAC), inflammatory markers (for TB-500), or liver function tests (for Melanotan II).

2. **Regular Checkups:** Schedule regular follow-ups with your healthcare provider to evaluate effectiveness and safety. Tests can be done every 3 months or more frequently if any adverse symptoms appear.

3. **Symptom Journaling:** Keep a daily log of how you feel after taking your peptide supplements. Note any side effects, changes in energy levels, sleep quality, appetite, or mood changes.
4. **Dosage Adjustments:** Based on feedback from blood tests and symptom journals, your dosage might need to be adjusted. Start with a lower dose and gradually increase as tolerated.

Monitoring Chart Example:

PEPTIDE	BASELINE TEST	COMMON SIDE EFFECTS	FOLLOW-UP INTERVAL
BPC-157	Digestive Health	Dizziness, Digestive Upset	Every 3 months
CJC-1295 with DAC	Hormone Levels	Fatigue, Headaches	Every 3 months
GHRP-6	Hormone Levels	Increased Hunger	Every 3 months
Thymosin Beta-4 (TB-500)	Inflammatory Markers	Redness at Injection Site	Every 3 months
Melanotan II	Liver Function	Nausea, Flushing	Monthly
Epithalon	General Wellness	Gastrointestinal Disturbances	Every 3 months

CHAPTER 4

ETHICAL AND LEGAL CONSIDERATIONS

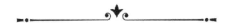

Regulatory Status of Peptides

Regulating peptides involves balancing safety, efficacy, and accessibility. Various governmental agencies oversee this process within their respective jurisdictions.

United States

In the United States, the Food and Drug Administration (FDA) is the primary body responsible for regulating peptides used for therapeutic purposes.

1. **Approval Process:** Peptides intended for clinical use must undergo rigorous preclinical and clinical testing. The Investigational New Drug (IND) application is the first step, allowing for initial trials in humans. Following successful trials, a New Drug Application (NDA) or a Biologics License Application (BLA) must be submitted for full market approval.
2. **Regulations:** The FDA classifies therapeutic peptides based on their complexity and production process—they may fall under small-molecule drugs or biologics, following specific regulatory pathways accordingly.

PHASE	DESCRIPTION

Preclinical	Laboratory and animal studies to assess safety and efficacy.
IND Submission	Application to conduct human clinical trials.
Clinical Trials	Human testing in phased trials (Phase I-III).
NDA/BLA Submission	Application for marketing approval based on trial data.

European Union

The European Medicines Agency (EMA) regulates peptides within the EU through a centralized procedure to ensure consistency across member states.

1. **Approval Process:** Manufacturers must submit a Marketing Authorization Application (MAA) that includes comprehensive preclinical and clinical study data.
2. **Orphan Designation:** For rare diseases, peptides can qualify for orphan designation, providing benefits like reduced fees and market exclusivity.

AGENCY	KEY FUNCTION
EMA	Overall regulation in EU
EMA	Committee for Medicinal Products for Human Use review panel.

Japan

The Pharmaceuticals and Medical Devices Agency (PMDA) oversees peptide regulation in Japan.

1. **Approval Process:** Similar to the FDA's procedure involving clinical trials backed by robust scientific evidence.
2. **Regulatory Pathway:** After successful trials, a New Drug Application (NDA) is filed with PMDA for review.

Other Regions

Different regions have their unique frameworks:

1. **Canada:** Health Canada oversees peptide regulation through its Biologics and Genetic Therapies Directorate.
2. **Australia:** The Therapeutic Goods Administration (TGA) manages peptide approval with guidelines similar to those in Western countries.

Understanding the regulatory environment for peptides is important for harnessing their full potential in extending human life span and enhancing quality of life. Adhering to strict regulatory requirements ensures that these powerful molecules are both safe and effective for public use.

Ethical Use of Peptides

The use of peptides has many benefits. However, it's important to consider the ethics of using them. Ethical use means keeping patients safe, being fair, getting clear permission from patients, and following rules set by authorities.

Patient safety must be a priority when considering peptide therapies. Peptides can offer significant health benefits, from improved skin elasticity to enhanced muscle growth and cognitive function. However, ensuring these treatments are safe involves rigorous clinical trials and ongoing monitoring. Researchers and healthcare providers must fully understand the short and long-term effects of peptide use on the human body before administering them to patients.

Another important issue is making sure everyone can access peptide treatments fairly. Often, new medical treatments are only available to rich people. It's important to make peptides affordable and available to many people, not just the wealthy. This involves pushing for policies that ensure these treatments are inclusive for everyone.

Informed consent is also very important in peptide treatment. Patients should know what peptides are, how they work, their benefits, and any possible risks before starting treatment. This requires clear communication between doctors and patients. Medical professionals must make sure that patients receive all necessary information in simple terms, without confusing medical language.

Regulatory compliance cannot be overlooked when discussing the ethical use of peptides. Regulatory bodies like the FDA (Food and Drug Administration) in the United States have stringent requirements for approving new therapies and treatments. These regulations ensure that any new substance introduced into the market has been adequately tested for safety and efficacy. Healthcare providers should adhere strictly to these regulations and only use approved peptides in their practices.

Furthermore, there is an ethical obligation to avoid misuse or abuse of peptide therapies. For instance, athletes might seek peptide treatments for unfair performance enhancement rather than remedial health benefits. This could lead to health complications if used improperly or without medical supervision. Establishing clear guidelines on what constitutes appropriate use versus misuse is essential in promoting responsible application.

Another aspect worth mentioning is the importance of ongoing education for both healthcare providers and patients regarding peptide therapies. The field of peptide research is continuously evolving with new discoveries about their capabilities and limits. Continuous professional development ensures healthcare providers remain updated on best practices while educating patients helps them make informed decisions about their treatments.

Finally, there should be an emphasis on global collaboration concerning peptide research and application to standardize practices across borders. Different countries may have varied regulatory frameworks; thus international cooperation can help harmonize standards ensuring consistency in how peptides are used ethically worldwide.

Legal Aspects in Different Regions

The rules and regulations about peptides use are different depending on where you are. It's important for both doctors and patients to know these legal guidelines. Understanding these laws can help ensure that treatments are safe and effective. In some areas, peptides are strictly controlled, while in others, they may be more freely used. Knowing the legal requirements can prevent potential legal issues and ensure that treatments comply with regional laws. This awareness is crucial for safe medical practice and patient safety.

1. **United States:** In the United States, peptide regulations fall under the purview of the Food and Drug Administration (FDA). The FDA categorizes peptides under various classifications depending on their

intended use—such as for cosmetic or therapeutic purposes. Approved therapeutic peptides must undergo rigorous testing and clinical trials to ensure safety and efficacy. It's worth noting that while there are FDA-approved peptides, a significant number are available only through research purposes, meaning they cannot be legally prescribed by healthcare providers.

2. **European Union:** The European Union (EU) has a more centralized regulatory framework managed by the European Medicines Agency (EMA). Like the FDA, the EMA mandates stringent clinical trials to bring new peptides to market. However, individual member countries within the EU may have additional regulations that could impact how peptides are distributed and used. One notable aspect is the EU's focus on quality control; peptides must meet high Pharmaceutical Good Manufacturing Practice (GMP) standards before they can even be subjected to clinical testing.

3. **Canada:** In Canada, Health Canada is responsible for regulating medical peptides. The country has stringent rules similar to those of its southern neighbor, focusing primarily on patient safety. Market approval involves numerous phases of clinical testing. Peptides used for research purposes are generally more accessible, but they need to adhere to specific compliance guidelines that ensure they're not used clinically without proper authorization.

4. **Australia:** The Therapeutic Goods Administration (TGA) handles peptide regulation in Australia. This agency enforces comprehensive guidelines requiring robust clinical evidence before any medical peptide can be approved for therapeutic use. Like other regions, Australia allows for research-grade peptides but with clear restrictions to prevent misuse in clinical settings. Compounding pharmacies can formulate certain peptide medications but must comply with TGA's specific compounding regulations.

5. **Asia:** Peptide regulations across Asia show considerable variability due to differing national policies and levels of regulatory rigor. For example, Japan's Pharmaceuticals and Medical Devices Agency (PMDA) closely mirrors Western regulatory frameworks by demanding exhaustive clinical trials for peptide approval. On the other hand, countries like China have been less stringent historically but are moving towards tighter regulations due to increasing quality control concerns. India's approach features a blend of western-style regulation and more flexible guidelines which attracts global pharmaceutical companies but necessitates clear compliance.

6. **Middle East:** In Middle Eastern nations like the United Arab Emirates (UAE) and Saudi Arabia, peptide regulatory frameworks are continuously evolving. Agencies such as Saudi Food & Drug Authority (SFDA) have started aligning more closely with international standards like those of the FDA and EMA. There remains a degree of flexibility in how these substances can be used therapeutically or cosmetically; however, authorities are increasingly cracking down on non-compliant entities to safeguard public health.

7. **Russia:** The Russian Federation has its unique set of guidelines managed by agencies like Roszdravnadzor (Federal Service for Surveillance in Healthcare). The regulatory landscape can be complex due to overlapping jurisdictions regarding medical oversight and drug enforcement agencies. Unlike some Western counterparts, Russia's approval processes may involve shorter clinical trials depending on expedited pathways designed to fast-track medical innovations like peptides.

8. **South America**: Peptide regulation across South America is diverse; Brazil's National Health Surveillance Agency (ANVISA) has perhaps one of the most structured systems resembling European frameworks with detailed protocols for approval and quality control. Conversely, smaller nations may lack comprehensive regulatory structures making it riskier navigating their legal landscapes when procuring or using peptides.

Sourcing High-Quality Peptides

Given the significant role of Peptides, it is essential to source high-quality peptides, especially when they are used for therapeutic purposes. Here, we discuss the main considerations and steps you should take to ensure that you are getting the best peptides available.

What Makes a Peptide High-Quality?

A high-quality peptide meets various criteria that ensure its efficacy and safety. Here are some key factors to consider:

1. **Purity:** High-quality peptides should have high purity levels, typically above 95%. The higher the purity, the fewer impurities which can affect the peptide's functionality.
2. **Stability:** The peptide should be stable at room temperature and have a long shelf-life without degrading.
3. **Source:** It is important to know where and how the peptide was synthesized. Good manufacturing practices (GMP) certified labs are preferable.
4. **Formulation:** Check whether the peptide is in the right form for your intended use (e.g., powdered form, pre-mixed solution).
5. **Testing:** A reputable supplier will provide Certificate of Analysis (CoA) and other documentation showing testing results for purity and identification.

Reliable Sources for Sourcing Peptides

Finding a reliable source can be challenging but here are a few tips:

1. **Reputable Suppliers:** Choose suppliers with positive reviews, testimonials, and established histories in the industry.
2. **GMP Certified Labs:** Ensure that the peptides come from labs following good manufacturing practices to guarantee highest quality standards.
3. **Transparent Documentation:** Vendors should provide full transparency regarding testing results such as Certificates of Analysis and third-party lab tests.

Practical Tips for Ensuring You Get the Best Product

1. **Research Thoroughly:** Before purchasing a peptide, research different brands and their reputations within user communities.
2. **Check Reviews and Testimonials:** Look at customer feedback on forums or product review sites to gauge effectiveness and reliability.
3. **Verify Authenticity of CoAs:** Ensure that any provided Certificates of Analysis are legitimate by cross-referencing with an independent lab if possible.
4. **Communication with Supplier:** Contact suppliers directly with any questions or concerns about their products' quality or sourcing methods.

EXAMPLE COMPARISON OF PEPTIDE SUPPLIERS

SUPPLIER	PURITY	GMP CERTIFIED	TESTING DOCUMENTATION	CUSTOMER REVIEWS
Supplier A	98%	Yes	Comprehensive CoA	Excellent
Supplier B	95%	No	Basic purity info	Mixed
Supplier C	99%	Yes	Full third-party test	Very Good

Future of Peptide Regulations

Currently, peptides fall under various regulatory bodies depending on their use—be it therapeutic, cosmetic, or as supplements. Regulatory bodies like the Food and Drug Administration (FDA) in the United States, the European Medicines Agency (EMA), and other global regulators are tasked with ensuring that these substances are both safe and effective for consumers.

One reason peptide regulations will need to evolve is their expanding application in personalized medicine. Peptides can be tailored to an individual's genetic makeup, offering treatments that are more effective and have fewer side effects compared to traditional drugs. This shift towards personalized medicine means that regulatory frameworks must adapt to evaluate peptides on a case-by-case basis. These frameworks need to account for variations in manufacturing processes, dosing requirements, and potential long-term effects specific to different patient populations.

Another important factor driving regulatory changes is the rise of biotechnology firms producing an ever-increasing variety of peptide-based treatments. The regulatory landscape must keep pace with these innovations to ensure that new peptides are thoroughly tested for efficacy and safety before reaching the market. This may involve creating specific guidelines for clinical trials that are focused on peptides, which could streamline the approval process without compromising safety standards.

The intersection of peptides with sports and athletics also presents unique regulatory challenges. Performance-enhancing drugs have long been a contentious issue in sports, and peptides are no exception. To maintain fair play, organizations like the World Anti-Doping Agency (WADA) continuously update their lists of banned substances. As peptide therapies evolve, so too must the methods for detecting and regulating their use in sports. Advanced testing techniques will be necessary to distinguish between legitimate medical treatments and those used illicitly to gain a competitive edge.

Moreover, public awareness and demand for wellness applications involving peptides are on the rise. Many over-the-counter products claim various benefits, from muscle building to anti-aging properties. Regulatory bodies face the challenge of differentiating legitimate products from those making unverified or exaggerated claims. Rigorous testing and clear labeling will be essential to protect consumers from ineffective or potentially harmful products.

Global collaboration is another crucial element in shaping the future of peptide regulations. Peptide developments do not occur in isolation; they involve scientists, manufacturers, and regulators from around the world. International bodies may need to coordinate more closely to harmonize regulations across different countries, ensuring that safety standards are maintained universally while facilitating easier access to beneficial treatments.

Additionally, advances in digital health technologies such as electronic health records (EHRs) and wearable devices can support better monitoring of peptide usage and its effects on patients over time. These technological tools can provide valuable data that help refine regulatory practices by offering real-world insights into how peptides are used and their outcomes.

CHAPTER 5

CONCLUSION AND RESOURCES

As we conclude our *"Book 1: PEPTIDE ESSENTIALS"*, let's reflect on the journey we've taken together. We've explored the immense potential of peptides, their benefits, and how they can be integrated into your daily life for improved health and well-being. Let's briefly summarize key points and provide resources for those interested in furthering their knowledge about peptides.

Peptides have shown promising results in various aspects of health, including anti-aging, muscle growth, recovery, cognitive function, and overall vitality. Their ability to signal cellular activity makes them powerful tools in enhancing bodily functions naturally. By understanding how peptides work and applying this knowledge correctly, individuals can significantly improve their health outcomes.

Getting Started with Peptides

For those new to peptides, the first step is education. Understanding what peptides are and how they operate within the body is crucial. Start simple:

1. **Consult Professionals:** Always consult with healthcare providers or specialists before starting any peptide regimen. They can provide personalized advice based on your health needs.
2. **Start Small:** Begin with well-known and commonly used peptides like BPC-157 for healing or CJC-1295 for growth hormone release.
3. **Monitor Results:** Keep track of your progress by noting any changes in your health, energy levels, or physical appearance.
4. **Safety First:** Ensure you're purchasing peptides from reputable sources to avoid counterfeit products.

Continuing Education

Learning about peptides doesn't stop after you've read this book. The field is constantly evolving with new research findings and practical applications. Here are some ways to continue your education:

1. **Scientific Journals:** Read journals and studies on peptide research. Websites like PubMed offer a plethora of articles on various peptides and their effects.
2. **Online Courses:** Enroll in online courses or webinars about peptide therapy offered by credible institutions or professionals in the field.
3. **Books & Publications:** Stay updated with the latest books on peptide therapy written by experts.
4. **Professional Associations:** Join professional groups or associations focused on peptide research and application.
5. **Conferences & Seminars:** Attend conferences and seminars to learn from leading professionals in the peptide industry.
6. **Networking:** Engage with other professionals or enthusiasts who share an interest in peptide therapy. Online forums and social media groups can be valuable resources for sharing experiences and knowledge.

Trusted Sources for Peptides

Obtaining high-quality peptides from reputable sources is crucial for ensuring safety and efficacy. Here are some trusted suppliers known for their rigorous standards:

1. **BioTech Peptides:** Known for their comprehensive range of research-grade peptides that strictly comply with industry standards. Each product is lab-tested for purity and potency.
2. **Peptide Sciences:** Renowned for providing pharmaceutical-grade peptides with a commitment to transparency and third-party testing.
3. **PureRawz:** Offers a variety of peptides with certificates of analysis available to confirm their quality and purity.
4. **Blue Sky Peptide:** Specializes in a range of peptides used in laboratory research with an emphasis on quality control.

When purchasing peptides, always ensure the supplier provides documentation regarding the peptide's composition, purity level, and manufacturing process. It's also advisable to consult healthcare professionals before beginning any peptide supplementation regimen to ensure it aligns with your health goals and needs.

Supporting Scientific Literature

The efficacy of peptides is backed by extensive scientific research. Here are some key studies that support the therapeutic potential of peptides:

1. **Clinical Applications of Peptides in Medicine (Journal of Clinical Endocrinology & Metabolism):** This study discusses how different peptides are utilized in clinical settings across various treatments including hormone regulation, metabolic disorders, and immune modulation.
2. **Peptides as Therapeutics: Current Approaches (Nature Reviews Drug Discovery):** Offers a comprehensive overview of how peptide-based therapeutics are developed, their advantages over conventional drugs, and current clinical trials data.

3. **Regenerative Effects of Peptides in Human Physiology (Frontiers in Endocrinology):** Highlights research on how specific peptides can promote regeneration at the cellular level, supporting tissue repair and healthy aging.
4. **Peptide-based Strategies Against Cardiovascular Diseases (Cardiovascular Research):** Explores the role of certain peptides in protecting heart health through mechanisms such as improving blood vessel function and reducing inflammation.
5. **Role of Peptides in Skin Health (Journal of Dermatological Science):** Examines how peptides contribute to skin rejuvenation by enhancing collagen production and improving skin elasticity.

Community and Forums

Engaging with communities and forums can be an invaluable resource when learning about peptides. These platforms allow you to gain insights from others' experiences, stay updated on the latest trends, and get answers to any questions you might have.

1. **Reddit:** Websites like Reddit have specific subreddits dedicated to peptide discussions where users share experiences, ask questions, and provide peer-reviewed advice.

   a. *r/Peptides:* This is one of the largest forums discussing everything related to peptides. Users share their experiences, ask questions, discuss suppliers, and provide feedback on different peptide protocols.
   b. *r/Nootropics:* While primarily focused on cognitive enhancers, this subreddit often covers peptides as well. It's a great place to find discussions on how certain peptides might affect cognitive functions.

Be cautious as not all advice on public forums is vetted by professionals. Always cross-check information received here with credible sources or professionals.

2. **Forums:**

   a. *Professional Muscle Forum:* This forum has a dedicated section for peptide discussions where experienced bodybuilders and fitness enthusiasts share their knowledge about using peptides for muscle building, fat loss, and overall health enhancement.
   b. *Peptide Forum:* Hosting specialized discussions ranging from details about specific peptides to symptoms experienced by users. It's an excellent resource for anyone new to using peptides or looking for more nuanced advice.

3. **Social Media Groups:** Facebook hosts numerous groups focused on peptide therapy where members discuss protocols, share success stories, troubleshoot problems, and recommend sources. Join groups with active moderation to ensure discussions stay relevant and misinformation is minimized.

   a. *Peptides & SARMs Discussion Group:* A private group focused on both education and user experiences regarding various peptide uses.
   b. *Real Peptide Group:* Another accessible group where members discuss sourcing, efficacy, side effects, etc.

4. **Dedicated Peptide Websites:** Some websites offer a comprehensive array of resources on peptides including articles, user guides, forums, and expert Q&A sections. Examples include websites like PeptideSciences.com or Peptides.org which also host community forums for user interaction.

BOOK 2
PEPTIDE PROTOCOLS

CHAPTER 1

TARGETED STRATEGIES FOR HEALTH

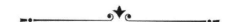

Health requires careful strategies to maintain. Targeted health strategies, like using peptide therapy, help improve overall well-being. Peptides are short chains of amino acids that are important for many biological processes. These strategies allow for a personalized approach to healthcare, addressing specific needs with tailored interventions.

One benefit of targeted strategies is the enhancement of treatment efficacy. By focusing on specific health issues, these strategies provide direct solutions and reduce side effects. They also support preventive healthcare by identifying and addressing health issues early, which can prevent diseases from developing or worsening. This helps lower healthcare costs and improves quality of life.

Targeted health strategies also empower individuals to take control of their health with personalized plans. These plans help people make informed decisions based on their unique needs. This leads to a better commitment to maintaining health. Overall, targeted health strategies are essential for effective disease management, prevention, and personalization of healthcare, leading to better long-term wellness.

Peptides for Longevity

As we get older, our bodies encounter various problems, like decreased cell function and higher chances of chronic illnesses. Among many methods to promote a longer life, peptides stand out as a beneficial group of substances. Peptides are small chains made of amino acids and are crucial in many bodily processes. They can be used to enhance health and potentially extend our lifespan. In this chapter, we will look at different types of peptides that help with longevity, explain how they work, and discuss ways to use them in daily life.

Several peptides show significant potential in promoting longevity. Here are some key categories:

1. Growth Hormone Secretagogues (GHS):

Example: Sermorelin

Function: Stimulates the pituitary gland to produce more growth hormone (GH). Increased GH levels can improve muscle mass, reduce body fat, and enhance overall vitality.

2. Thymic Peptides:

Example: Thymosin Alpha-1

Function: Enhances immune function by promoting T-cell production and activity. A robust immune system is crucial for fighting infections and diseases associated with aging.

3. Mitochondrial Peptides:

Example: MOTS-c

Function: Promotes mitochondrial health and energy production. Healthy mitochondria are essential for cellular energy and reducing oxidative stress, which contributes to aging.

4. Neuroprotective Peptides:

Example: Cerebrolysin

Function: Supports brain health by promoting neuron growth and repair. Protecting cognitive function is vital as we age, reducing the risk of neurodegenerative diseases like Alzheimer's.

Mechanisms Behind Peptide Actions

Peptides work through several mechanisms to promote longevity:

1. **Cell Signaling:** Peptides act as signaling molecules that bind to specific receptors on cell surfaces, triggering various biological responses.

Example: GHS peptides stimulate receptors in the pituitary gland to release growth hormone.

2. **Gene Expression Modulation:** Some peptides can influence gene expression, turning on or off certain genes that play a role in aging.

Example: MOTS-c can alter the expression of genes involved in mitochondrial function.

3. **Immune System Support:** Certain peptides boost the immune system's ability to combat pathogens and clear damaged cells.

Example: Thymosin Alpha-1 enhances the activity of T-cells responsible for identifying and destroying infected or dysfunctional cells.

4. **Anti-Inflammatory Effects:** Chronic inflammation is a significant contributing factor to aging-related diseases.

Example: Some peptides have anti-inflammatory properties that help minimize tissue damage over time.

Practical Applications

Incorporating peptides into a longevity regimen requires careful consideration and professional guidance:

1. **Consultation with Healthcare Professionals:** Always seek advice from healthcare providers experienced in peptide therapy. Personalized peptide protocols based on individual health status can maximize benefits and minimize risks.

2. **Administration Methods:** Common methods include injection, oral supplements, or topical creams. Each method has different absorption rates and efficacy; discuss options with your healthcare provider.

3. **Monitoring Progress:** Regular follow-ups with healthcare providers ensure that peptide therapy is effective and adjustments can be made as needed. Monitoring biomarkers like hormone levels, immune function markers, and mitochondrial health indicators helps track progress.

4. **Combining with Lifestyle Practices:** Peptides are most effective when used alongside healthy lifestyle choices. Regular physical activity, a balanced diet, adequate sleep, and stress management can amplify the benefits of peptide therapy.

Peptides offer a promising approach to promoting longevity by targeting key biological processes involved in aging. When combined with professional guidance and a healthy lifestyle, peptides can significantly enhance health span and quality of life as we age.

Peptides for Brain Health

The human brain is important for everything we do, from basic tasks like breathing to thinking complex thoughts. As we get older, keeping our brain working well is essential. Peptides can help with this. hey help neurons talk to each other, protect brain cells from harm, and even help create new brain cells. For example, some peptides can improve memory and learning by making sure that different parts of the brain work well together. Others can act like a shield, keeping brain cells safe from damage caused by things like stress or toxins. Additionally, some peptides encourage the growth of new neurons, which is essential for maintaining a healthy and active brain.

They can also reduce inflammation in the brain, which is linked to diseases like Alzheimer's. Peptides occur naturally in foods like fish, meat, and dairy, but they can also be made in labs for supplements. Using peptides for brain health may help keep our minds sharp as we age. Let's explore a few specific peptides that are known for supporting brain health.

1. **Cerebrolysin:** Cerebrolysin is a peptide mixture derived from pig brain proteins. It has been widely studied for its neuroprotective properties. Research suggests that Cerebrolysin promotes neuron survival, enhances neuronal communication, and even stimulates dendrite growth (branches of neurons that receive signals). This makes it particularly promising for treating neurodegenerative diseases like Alzheimer's and Parkinson's.

2. **Selank**: Selank is a synthetic peptide that mimics the effects of tuftsin, a natural immunomodulatory peptide found in the body. Studies have shown that Selank can reduce anxiety and enhance cognitive functions such as memory and learning. It achieves this by modulating the balance of neurotransmitters in the brain, reducing inflammation, and promoting neurogenesis.

3. **Semax**: Semax is another synthetic peptide, originally developed in Russia for treating stroke victims. It has been shown to offer neuroprotective benefits and improve cognitive function by enhancing brain-derived neurotrophic factor (BDNF) levels. BDNF is crucial for supporting neuron survival and growth, making Semax a valuable tool for enhancing overall brain health.

4. **PE-22-28 (also known as P21)**: PE-22-28 is a fragment derived from an anti-aging peptide called Epitalon. Research indicates that PE-22-28 can promote neural cell proliferation and reduce oxidative stress in the brain. These benefits have led researchers to explore its potential for mitigating age-related cognitive decline.

5. **Noopept**: Noopept isn't technically a peptide but is worth mentioning due to its similar functions and widespread use as a neuroprotective agent. It has been shown to boost memory, focus, and overall cognitive performance by increasing levels of certain neurotransmitters like acetylcholine and glutamate.

Each peptide works through different mechanisms to benefit the brain:

1. **Neuroprotection:** Many peptides provide a protective effect against various forms of damage including oxidative stress and acute injury.
2. **Neurogenesis:** Some peptides like Selank encourage the growth of new neurons.
3. **Neurotransmitter Balance:** Several peptides help regulate neurotransmitters like dopamine, serotonin, and acetylcholine, which are crucial for mood stability and cognitive functions.

The use of these peptides generally involves administration via injections or nasal sprays due to their inability to withstand the acidic environment of the stomach if taken orally. However, research continues into oral formulations that could offer more convenient alternatives in the future. Peptides have shown promise not only in clinical settings but also as nootropic supplements aimed at improving everyday cognitive functions among healthy individuals.

Peptides for Physical Performance

Improving physical performance often involves enhancing the body's natural functions. Peptides have proven to be useful in this area. Peptides work in various ways to enhance physical abilities. They can help increase muscle growth, improve recovery times, and even support fat loss. Some peptides stimulate the release of growth hormone, which is essential for muscle development and repair. Others help reduce inflammation and promote faster healing of injuries.

Peptides and Muscle Growth

One of the most extensively researched and utilized peptides in sports and fitness is Growth Hormone-Releasing Peptide (GHRP). GHRPs stimulate the release of growth hormone from the pituitary gland, which plays a pivotal role in muscle growth and repair. Increased levels of growth hormone can lead to enhanced muscle protein synthesis, faster recovery times, and increased lean body mass.

Another prominent peptide is the CJC-1295, which also promotes muscle growth by increasing endogenous human growth hormone levels. When combined with proper training and nutrition, these peptides can significantly amplify muscle development.

Peptides for Fat Loss

In addition to building muscle, maintaining an optimal body composition is vital for peak physical performance. Peptides such as Melanotan II have been shown to assist in fat loss by increasing metabolism and promoting fat oxidation. Melanotan II works by stimulating melanocortin receptors in the brain, which in turn regulates appetite and increases energy expenditure.

Other peptides like Fragment 176-191 specifically target adipose tissue by mimicking the way natural growth hormones control fat metabolism without affecting other metabolic processes. This specificity makes Fragment 176-191 particularly attractive for athletes aiming to reduce body fat while preserving lean muscle mass.

Enhanced Recovery

Effective recovery protocols are crucial for maintaining consistent training intensity and preventing injuries. TB-500 (Thymosin Beta-4) is a peptide known for its ability to promote healing and reduce inflammation. It helps by stimulating cell migration and new blood vessel formation at injury sites, accelerating recovery from physical exertion or trauma.

BPC-157 (Body Protection Compound) is another peptide widely recognized for its regenerative properties. Research indicates that BPC-157 can heal tendons, ligaments, muscles, nerves, and even gastrointestinal tissues. This broad spectrum of healing capabilities makes it invaluable not only for athletes but also for anyone seeking improved recovery from strenuous activities.

Enhancing Endurance

Cardiovascular performance and endurance can be enhanced with peptides such as Aicar (Aminoimidazole Carboxamide Ribonucleotide). Aicar stimulates AMP-activated protein kinase (AMPK), which plays a crucial role in cellular energy homeostasis. By activating AMPK, Aicar enhances glucose uptake by cells and increases fatty acid oxidation in muscles, thus improving endurance levels. Moreover, BPC-157 has also shown potential benefits in enhancing endurance due to its vascular healing properties, supporting better blood flow during prolonged physical activity.

Peptides for Improved Joint Health

Joint health is critical for athletes and those engaged in regular physical activity. Peptides such as IGF-1 LR3 (Insulin-like Growth Factor 1 Long R3) can play a significant role in improving joint health by promoting cartilage repair and regeneration. This peptide helps increase the production of synovial fluid, which lubricates joints and reduces friction during movement.

Additionally, the peptide known as Thymosin Beta-4 (TB-500) has anti-inflammatory properties that can alleviate joint pain and promote healing of connective tissues. By reducing inflammation and supporting tissue repair, TB-500 helps maintain joint health even under strenuous physical activities.

Enhanced Sleep Quality

Quality sleep is essential for physical performance and overall recovery. Peptides like DSIP (Delta Sleep Inducing Peptide) can help enhance sleep quality by promoting deep, restful sleep. Deep sleep is crucial as it is the phase during which most tissue repair and growth occur. Improved sleep quality aids in better recovery, enhanced mood, and increased energy levels.

PEPTIDE	MAIN BENEFITS	MECHANISM OF ACTION	TYPICAL USAGE
GHRP	Muscle growth and recovery	Stimulates release of growth hormone	Combined with resistance training
CJC-1295	Increased muscle mass	Enhances endogenous HGH secretion	Cycled with periods off
Melanotan II	Fat loss	Stimulates melanocortin receptors	Moderated doses
Fragment 176-191	Targeted fat reduction	Mimics GH role in fat metabolism	Gradual dose increases
TB-500	Enhanced recovery	Promotes cellular healing and reduces inflammation	Post-injury supplementation
BPC-157	Accelerated healing of tissues	Promotes cellular repair and blood vessel growth	Post-injury supplementation
Aicar	Improved endurance	Activates AMPK, enhancing energy utilization	Pre-event preparation
IGF-1 LR3	Joint health	Promotes cartilage repair and synovial fluid production	Recovery cycles
DSIP	Enhanced sleep quality	Induces deep sleep	Before bedtime

Using peptides can help improve physical performance in several ways. They support muscle growth, aid in fat loss, speed up recovery, and assist with joint health. Adding the right peptides to your training routine can boost strength, endurance, and overall athletic abilities.

Peptides for Immune Boosting

The immune system serves as our body's defense against harmful invaders like bacteria, viruses, and other pathogens. One of the promising ways to enhance this defense mechanism is through the use of peptides, which are short chains of amino acids that play crucial roles in regulating various physiological processes. Peptides can modulate the immune system in several key ways:

1. **Activation of Immune Cells:** Certain peptides help in the activation and proliferation of immune cells such as T-cells and B-cells, which are essential for adaptive immunity.
2. **Anti-Inflammatory Properties:** Some peptides reduce inflammation by inhibiting the production of pro-inflammatory cytokines.
3. **Antimicrobial Activity:** Specific peptides can directly kill bacteria, viruses, and fungi, providing an immediate line of defense.
4. **Tissue Repair:** Peptides assist in repairing damaged tissues, helping to maintain a strong immune barrier.

Key Immune-Boosting Peptides

1. **Thymosin Alpha-1:** This peptide is derived from the thymus gland and has been shown to enhance the function of T-cells, which are crucial for adaptive immunity. Thymosin Alpha-1 plays a role in augmenting the body's natural defenses against bacterial, fungal, and viral infections. It also has potential benefits in treating conditions like hepatitis B and C, and it's being researched as a supportive treatment for various cancers.

2. **LL-37:** LL-37 is an antimicrobial peptide that helps fight pathogens by breaking down their cell membranes. It not only has direct antimicrobial actions but also modulates immune responses, making it more effective in combatting infections. Research suggests that LL-37 can be instrumental in treating chronic infections and promoting wound healing.

3. **IKK Beta-TLR4 Inhibitor Peptide (C34):** This peptide works by inhibiting inflammatory pathways within the immune system. Chronic inflammation can weaken the immune response over time, so using a peptide like C34 can help strengthen overall immunity by reducing excessive inflammatory processes.

Several studies have documented the effectiveness of these peptides in enhancing immune function:

1. A clinical trial involving Thymosin Alpha-1 showed increased survival rates among patients with severe sepsis.
2. Research indicates that LL-37 promotes healing in chronic wound conditions such as diabetic foot ulcers by enhancing local immune responses.
3. Preclinical studies with IKK Beta-TLR4 Inhibitor Peptide (C34) demonstrate reduced inflammation and improved outcomes in autoimmune disease models.

PEPTIDE	SOURCE	MECHANISM OF ACTION	APPLICATIONS
Thymosin Alpha-1	Thymus Gland	Enhances T-cell function	Viral infections (e.g., hepatitis), cancer therapy support
LL-37	Human Host	Direct antimicrobial action	Chronic infections, wound healing
IKK Beta-TLR4 Inhibitor	Synthetic	Inhibits inflammatory pathways	Autoimmune diseases

The potential of peptides to boost immune functions offers exciting possibilities for enhancing overall health and combating various diseases. Through modulation of T-cell activity, balancing cytokine levels, and direct antimicrobial actions, peptides such as Thymosin Alpha-1, LL-37, and IKK Beta-TLR4 Inhibitor provide promising strategies for fortifying our body's natural defenses. While further research is always valuable for deeper understanding and broader applications, current evidence strongly supports.

Peptides for Hormonal Balance

The human body relies on hormonal balance to maintain health and vitality. Hormones are chemical messengers that coordinate various functions in the body, influencing everything from mood to metabolism. Imbalances in hormone levels can lead to numerous health issues, including fatigue, weight gain, mood swings, and more serious conditions like diabetes and thyroid disorders. Fortunately, peptides offer a promising solution for those looking to balance their hormones naturally.

Peptides facilitate communication between cells and help regulate biological processes. When it comes to hormonal balance, certain peptides act as precursors or stimulants for hormone production, while others inhibit the production of excessive hormones. These peptides can be administered through various methods including oral supplements, injections, and transdermal patches.

Key Peptides for Hormonal Balance

1. **Growth Hormone-Releasing Peptides (GHRPs)**: GHRPs such as GHRP-2 and GHRP-6 stimulate the pituitary gland to release growth hormone (GH). An increase in GH levels can enhance metabolism, support muscle growth, improve energy levels, and contribute to overall well-being.
2. **Thymosin Alpha-1**: Thymosin Alpha-1 boosts immune function by influencing the thymus gland. While it mainly supports immunity, it also indirectly helps maintain a balanced hormonal environment by reducing stress on other endocrine glands.
3. **Corticotropin-Releasing Factor (CRF) Peptides**: CRF-related peptides work by targeting the adrenal glands to produce cortisol when needed while preventing overproduction that can lead to stress-related disorders. Proper cortisol levels are vital for managing stress responses without causing extended periods of high cortisol which can disrupt other hormonal functions.
4. **Kisspeptin**: Kisspeptin impacts reproductive hormones by influencing the secretion of Gonadotropin-Releasing Hormone (GnRH). This helps regulate menstrual cycles in women and sperm production in men by maintaining healthy levels of estrogen and testosterone.
5. **Melanotan II**: Melanotan II influences melanocyte-stimulating hormone (MSH), which can have a utility beyond skin darkening effects; it also has impacts on appetite regulation and lipid metabolism that indirectly contribute to a balanced hormonal state.

PEPTIDE	TARGET HORMONE	MECHANISM OF ACTION	APPLICATIONS
GHRP-2 / GHRP-6	Growth Hormone	Enhanced muscle growth; energy levels	Anti-aging; fitness support
Thymosin Alpha-1	Immune hormones	Improved immune response	Immune support
CRF-related peptides	Cortisol	Stress regulation; adrenal function	Stress management
Kisspeptin	GnRH	Regulation of reproductive hormones	Fertility; menstrual regularity
Melanotan II	MSH	Appetite control; lipid metabolism	Weight management

CHAPTER 2

DETAILED PROTOCOLS

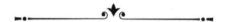

Detailed protocols are the backbone of successful peptide therapy. They ensure consistency, safety, and efficacy in treatments that aim to enhance longevity, vitality, and well-being. Without detailed instructions, the application of peptide protocols might vary widely, leading to unpredictable outcomes. Detailed protocols help in standardizing procedures so that every practitioner can achieve similar results, reducing the likelihood of errors or adverse effects.

Moreover, detailed protocols contribute to the reproducibility of scientific findings. When researchers document precise steps and conditions under which experiments are conducted, other scientists can replicate these experiments to verify results. This rigor is crucial for advancing our understanding of peptide therapies.

Another significant aspect is patient trust. Patients are more likely to adhere to treatment plans when they understand each step involved. Clear protocols provide a roadmap that guides both the practitioner and the patient through the process, ensuring all necessary actions are taken to maximize the benefits while minimizing risks. Lastly, detailed protocols serve as educational tools for new practitioners entering the field. They offer a comprehensive guide that takes one from beginner to expert, ensuring that knowledge is passed down accurately.

Protocol Design

Creating an effective peptide protocol begins with a deep understanding of the goals you aim to achieve. Whether it's enhancing vitality, extending longevity, or improving overall well-being, the design of your protocol needs to be meticulously planned and tailored to meet these objectives.

Clearly outline the specific goals for the peptide protocol. Are you looking to boost immunity, enhance muscle growth, improve cognitive function, or support joint health? Knowing the purpose will guide your choice of peptides and their combinations.

Research various peptides that align with your goals. Here are some common peptides and their functions:

1. **BPC-157:** Known for its healing properties and beneficial for joint health.
2. **HGH Fragment 176-191:** Often used for fat loss.
3. **CJC-1295:** Promotes muscle growth and recovery.
4. **Ipamorelin:** Helps with anti-aging and enhances muscle mass.

Dosage Calculation

The right dosage is crucial for the effectiveness and safety of peptide treatments. It should be based on your body weight, age, health, and specific needs. Here are some important points to consider:

1. Starting doses typically range from 0.5 mg to 1 mg per day.
2. The way you take it can change the dose needed. For example, under-the-skin injections might require a different dose compared to other methods.

PEPTIDE	LOW DOSE	MEDIUM DOSE	HIGH DOSE
BPC-157	100 mcg/day	250 mcg/day	500 mcg/day
HGH Frag 176-191	250 mcg/day	500 mcg/day	1 mg/day
CJC-1295 + DAC	300 mcg/week	600 mcg/week	1 mg/week
Ipamorelin	100 mcg/day	200 mcg/day	300 mcg/day

The timing of peptide administration can affect outcomes. Some peptides like Ipamorelin are best taken before sleep due to their growth hormone-releasing effects during sleep cycles. Others might need to be taken multiple times a day based on their half-life.

PEPTIDE	MORNING	AFTERNOON	EVENING
BPC-157			X (after meals)
HGH Frag 176-191	X (fasting)		X (before sleep)
CJC-1295 + DAC	X		
Ipamorelin			X

Administration Routes

The method of delivery can also influence effectiveness and compliance:

1. **Subcutaneous Injection:** Common for most peptide protocols.
2. **Oral/Sublingual:** Limited bioavailability but easier administration.
3. **Intranasal/Inhalation:** For specific peptides targeting the brain or nasopharyngeal regions.

Establishing cycle duration and necessary breaks helps prevent tolerance build-up and side effects. Typical cycle lengths can vary from a few weeks to several months. Including off-cycles or breaks can help maintain peptide effectiveness over time.

Monitoring Progress

Regular monitoring is essential for any peptide protocol. Document changes in physical health, lab results, and overall well-being:

1. Keep a journal to track dosage, administration times, side effects, and improvements.
2. Schedule regular blood tests to monitor biomarkers influenced by peptides like IGF-1 for growth hormone-related peptides.

Combining Peptides

Combining different peptides can enhance their synergistic effects but requires careful planning:

1. **Complementary Functions:** Choose peptides that complement each other's functions (e.g., combining a healing peptide like BPC-157 with a muscle growth peptide like CJC-1295).
2. **Avoid Overlapping Pathways:** Be cautious about combining peptides that target the same physiological pathways to reduce the risk of overstimulation and negative side effects.

Review and Feedback Loop

Establish a feedback loop for continuous improvement of your peptide protocol:

1. **Regular Reviews:** Set intervals (e.g., monthly) to review your journal entries and blood test results.
2. **Professional Feedback:** Discuss findings with your healthcare provider to make informed decisions about continuing or modifying the protocol.
3. **Stay Updated:** Keep abreast of new research and developments in peptide science to optimize your protocol over time.

Step-by-Step Instructions

To initiate your journey with peptide protocols, clear and concise step-by-step instructions are essential. This section offers detailed guidance to ensure effective and safe application, maximizing benefits for longevity, vitality, and well-being. Here is a comprehensive walkthrough on how to administer peptide protocols following a structured approach:

Step 1: Preparation

1. **Gather Materials:**

   ☐ Your selected peptide (vial)
   ☐ Bacteriostatic water (sterile water)
   ☐ Alcohol swabs

☐ Insulin syringes
☐ Disposable gloves
☐ Ampule breaker (if needed)

2. **Clean Workspace:** Ensure that you're working in a clean environment. Sanitize the surface you'll be using.

3. **Wash Hands:** Thoroughly wash your hands with soap and water before handling any materials.

Step 2: Reconstitution of Peptides

1. **Assess Vial:** Check the peptide vial for any damage or cloudiness, which may indicate contamination.

2. **Alcohol Swab:** Swab the top of the peptide vial and bacteriostatic water vial with an alcohol swab.

3. **Draw Bacteriostatic Water:** Use the insulin syringe to draw up the required amount of bacteriostatic water (typically 1-2 ml).

4. **Inject into Peptide Vial:** Slowly inject the bacteriostatic water into the peptide vial by letting it run down the side of the vial to minimize frothing.

5. **Gently Mix Solution:** Do not shake the vial; instead, gently swirl to mix until fully dissolved.

Step 3: Proper Storage

1. **Label Vials:** Label your reconstituted peptide vial with date and dosage information.

2. **Refrigeration:** Store peptides in a refrigerator at a temperature between 2-8°C (36-46°F).

3. **Avoid Light & Heat Exposure:** Protect from light by storing vials in their original packaging or a light-proof container.

Step 4: Administering Peptides

1. **Dosage Calculation and Draw Up Peptide Solution:** Calculate individual dosage based on protocol guidelines. Draw up calculated dose using an insulin syringe.

Weight (kg)	Dosage per Injection (mcg/kg)	Total Dose (mcg)
60	5	300
70	5	350
80	5	400

2. **Choose Injection Site:** Pinch skin to lift subcutaneous layer using clean gloves.

Common sites include:

☐ Subcutaneous fat on abdomen
☐ Thighs

3. **Disinfect Injection Site:** Use an alcohol swab to clean selected injection area in circular motions.

4. **Perform Injection:** Hold the syringe like a dart at a 45-degree angle. Insert syringe swiftly into pinched skin. Press plunger gently until complete dose injected. Dispose of needle safely in sharps container immediately after use.

Step 5: Post-Injection Care

1. **Observation Criteria & Symptom Monitoring:** Check injection site for redness, swelling, or irritation. Note overall physical response within hours/days post-injection and report unanticipated reactions immediately.

2. **Document Administered Doses:** Keep accurate records for each dose administered, including time/date plus specific doses used. Regular review helps manage protocols better while optimizing outcomes long-term.

Step 6: Safety and Compliance

1. **Use Consistent Hygiene Practices:** Always follow the same sanitary protocols to minimize the risk of contamination or infection.

2. **Regular Check-Ins:** Schedule regular check-ins with your healthcare provider to monitor progress and make any necessary adjustments to your protocol.

3. **Dispose of Medical Waste Properly:** Use a designated sharps container for disposing of needles and syringes to ensure safety.

4. **Adhere to Legal Guidelines:** Ensure that you are in compliance with any local laws or regulations regarding the use of peptides.

Step 7: Monitoring and Adjustments

1. **Track Progress:** Keep a detailed log of your injection schedule, dosages, and any effects observed. This will help you track your progress over time.

2. **Adjust Dosages if Necessary:** Based on your tracking and feedback from your healthcare provider, adjust dosages as needed to optimize results.

3. **Periodic Lab Tests:** Regular lab tests may be recommended to monitor peptide levels and overall health markers.

4. **Consult Healthcare Provider for Adjustments:** Work closely with your healthcare provider when making any changes to your protocol to ensure they are safe and effective.

SAMPLE DAILY LOG TEMPLATE					
DATE	**TIME**	**PEPTIDE USED**	**DOSE (MCG)**	**INJECTION SITE**	**NOTES**
DD-MM-YYYY	8 AM	Peptide X	300	Abdomen	No irritation observed
DD-MM-YYYY	8 AM	Peptide X	300	Thigh	Slight redness noted
DD-MM-YYYY	8 AM	Peptide X	300	Abdomen	Feeling increased energy

This detailed guide will assist you in safely and effectively administering peptide protocols, ensuring maximum benefits for longevity, vitality, and well-being. Always consult with a healthcare professional before starting any new treatment regimen.

Customizing Protocols

When it comes to improving health through peptide treatments, one-size-fits-all does not work. Each person is different, so it's important to make specific plans for each individual. Customizing peptide protocols means creating a plan that fits a person's unique body and goals. This approach helps achieve better results because it takes into account each person's specific needs. Customizing ensures that the treatment works best for each individual, improving their overall health and well-being.

Key Considerations for Customization

1. **Individual Health Profile**

   a. *Medical History:* Assess any pre-existing conditions, allergies, or previous responses to similar protocols.
   b. *Current Health Status:* Evaluate current physical condition, including recent lab tests and biomarkers.
   c. *Lifestyle Factors:* Consider diet, exercise regimen, sleep patterns, and stress levels.

2. **Goals and Outcomes**

   a. *Short-term Goals:* These may include immediate benefits like improved sleep quality or increased energy levels.
   b. *Long-term Goals:* Focus on sustained improvements like enhanced immune function or muscle mass gain.

3. **Peptide Types and Combinations**: Understanding which peptides serve specific roles is essential for customization. For instance:

   a. *Growth Hormone Secretagogues (GHS):* Targeted for muscle growth or fat loss.
   b. *Bioregulators:* Used for organ-specific regeneration.
   c. *Neurotropic Peptides:* Aimed at cognitive enhancement.

4. **Dosage and Administration** Dosages need to be tailored based on weight, age, and health status. Administration routes (e.g., subcutaneous injections vs. oral intake) should also be customized.

Customization Framework

To effectively customize a peptide protocol, follow these steps:

1. **Initial Consultation**: Meet with a healthcare provider to discuss medical history, existing conditions, and desired outcomes.
2. **Baseline Testing**: Conduct laboratory tests to determine baseline levels of hormones, biomarkers, and other relevant metrics.
3. **Protocol Design**: Select peptides based on the data collected from the initial consultation and baseline testing. Determine the optimal dosage and administration schedule.

4. **Trial Period**: Implement the protocol for a defined period (e.g., 4-6 weeks). Keep a detailed log of any changes in symptoms or side effects.

5. **Monitor and Adjust**: Conduct follow-up testing to assess the effectiveness of the protocol. Make necessary adjustments to dosage or peptide combinations based on results and feedback.

6. **Maintenance Phase**: Once optimized, transition to a maintenance dose or periodic cycling depending on goals.

Case Studies of Detailed Protocols

Now, we will examine two distinct case studies to understand how peptide protocols can be effectively utilized in real-world scenarios. These case studies will provide a clear, step-by-step walkthrough of the protocols designed for specific health conditions and goals. Through these examples, we aim to illustrate the practical application, potential benefits, and adjustments required to optimize results.

Case Study 1: Enhancing Muscle Recovery in Athletes

Subject Profile:

- ☐ *Name:* John D.
- ☐ *Age:* 28
- ☐ *Occupation:* Professional Athlete (Soccer Player)
- ☐ *Goal:* Accelerate muscle recovery and enhance performance

Background: John D. is a professional soccer player who experiences significant muscle fatigue and occasional injuries due to rigorous training and matches. His primary goal is to reduce recovery time between training sessions and improve overall muscle performance.

Protocol Design:

1. *Peptide Selection:* BPC-157 (Body Protection Compound) known for its healing properties and TB-500 for muscle recovery.
2. *Dosage:*
   - ☐ BPC-157: 250 mcg once daily
   - ☐ TB-500: 2 mg twice weekly
3. *Duration:* 8 weeks
4. *Administration Method:* Subcutaneous injections

Step-by-Step Instructions:

1. *Week 1-2:* Administer BPC-157 daily and TB-500 every three days. Monitor for any adverse reactions. Emphasize proper injection technique to minimize discomfort.
2. *Week 3-6:* Continue with the same dosage. Track progress using a daily journal focusing on recovery time, soreness levels, and overall performance. Increase hydration and maintain a balanced diet rich in proteins and essential nutrients.
3. *Week 7-8:* Assess muscle recovery improvements. Conduct physical tests such as sprints, endurance runs, and strength assessments. Compare results with baseline measurements taken before starting the protocol.

Results: John reported a noticeable reduction in muscle soreness within two weeks of starting the protocol. By the end of eight weeks, his recovery time between training sessions decreased by approximately 40%. Physical assessments showed a marked improvement in both endurance and strength.

Customizing Protocol: For John, minor adjustments were made based on his response to the peptides:

1. Increased BPC-157 dosage to 300 mcg daily during high-intensity training weeks.
2. Extended TB-500 administration by one month during peak soccer season for sustained benefits.

RECOVERY METRICS (BASELINE VS. POST PROTOCOL)		
METRIC	**BASELINE**	**AFTER PROTOCOL**
Muscle Soreness (1-10)	7	3
Recovery Time (hours)	48	28
Endurance Run (minutes)	15	18
Sprint Speed (seconds)	12	11

Case Study 2: Anti-Aging and Longevity Enhancement

Subject Profile:

- ☐ *Name:* Mary S.
- ☐ *Age:* 55
- ☐ *Occupation:* Retired Teacher
- ☐ *Goal:* Reduce signs of aging, enhance vitality, and improve overall well-being

Background: Mary S., a retired teacher, noticed signs of aging such as loss of skin elasticity, reduced energy levels, and some cognitive decline. Her objective was to address these issues through a comprehensive peptide protocol aimed at anti-aging and longevity enhancement.

Protocol Design:

1. *Peptide Selection:* Epithalon for anti-aging properties
2. *Dosage:*
   - ☐ Epithalon: 10 mg every day for 20 days
   - ☐ Thymalin: 10 mg every day for 20 days
3. *Duration:* Initial course of 20 days, with quarterly follow-ups
4. *Administration Method:* Subcutaneous injections

Step-by-Step Instructions:

1. *Days 1-20:* Administer Epithalon and Thymalin daily. Monitor for any side effects. Keep a log of skin condition, energy levels, and cognitive functioning.
2. *Follow-Up (Quarterly):* Repeat the 20-day course every three months. Evaluate overall well-being and adjust other lifestyle factors like diet and exercise accordingly.

Results: Mary experienced significant improvements in skin elasticity and overall vitality after one month. She reported feeling more energetic and noticed a reduction in minor cognitive issues.

Customizing Protocol: Based on Mary's progress, a few adjustments were made:

1. Increased the interval between courses to four months instead of three due to sustained benefits.
2. Complemented peptide therapy with a daily multivitamin.

WELLNESS METRICS (BASELINE VS. POST PROTOCOL)		
METRIC	**BASELINE**	**AFTER PROTOCOL**
Skin Elasticity (1-10)	4	7
Energy Levels (1-10)	5	8
Cognitive Function (1-10)	6	9

Protocol Evolution and Adaptation

Every protocol begins with an initial framework based on available scientific knowledge. Early peptide protocols were often rudimentary, based on limited understanding of how these compounds interact with body systems. As researchers observed outcomes and gathered more data, these protocols were refined. The iterative process started with basic steps, including dosing, administration routes, and frequency of use.

1. **Observational Data and Feedback Loops:** One essential aspect of protocol evolution is the systematic collection of observational data. Clinicians record patient responses to treatments—both positive effects and adverse reactions. This data forms feedback loops that help in refining the protocol. For example, a peptide initially administered subcutaneously might show improved results when given intramuscularly after reviewing patient feedback.

2. **Research and Technological Advancements:** Ongoing research continually supplies new insights into peptide efficacy, mechanisms of action, and safety profiles. Sophisticated technologies like high-throughput screening and computational biology allow for detailed study of peptides at molecular levels. These advancements facilitate identifying more effective peptides or new uses for existing ones. Consequently, protocols adapt to incorporate these insights, leading to more successful therapies.

3. **Individual Variability and Customization:** No two individuals respond identically to a given therapy due to genetic differences, environmental factors, lifestyle choices, and overall health conditions. Personalized medicine takes these variables into account by tailoring protocols on a case-by-case basis.

   a. *Genetic Testing:* In some cases, genetic screening can guide the selection of specific peptides or suggest dose adjustments.
   b. *Biomarker Monitoring:* Regular monitoring of biomarkers can indicate how well a patient is responding to treatment, allowing for real-time adjustments.
   c. *Patient Preferences:* Considerations like ease of administration or potential side effects can also influence protocol adaptation.

4. **Case Studies in Protocol Evolution**: The practice of evolving protocols can be illustrated with several examples:

    a. *Peptide X Protocol:* Initially prescribed thrice weekly at a standard dose, feedback indicated frequent reactions at the injection site. Researchers introduced a slow-release formulation that reduced administration frequency to once weekly without compromising effectiveness.

    b. *Peptide Y Protocol:* Originally recommended exclusively for muscle growth in athletes; observational studies showed it also significantly improved cognitive functions in elderly patients. The protocol was adapted to include cognitive enhancement as an additional benefit.

    c. *Peptide Z Protocol:* When this peptide was first used for metabolic syndrome management, some patients reported gastrointestinal discomfort. Adjustments such as splitting doses or changing administration times lessened side effects without impacting therapeutic outcomes.

5. **Continuous Improvement Cycle**: A cornerstone of effective protocol design is the commitment to ongoing improvement—a continuous cycle involving:

    a. *Routine Assessments:* Periodic review meetings among healthcare providers to discuss collected data and make necessary modifications.

    b. *Updated Training:* Regular training for practitioners on new findings and updated protocols ensures standardized implementation.

    c. *Patient Education:* Informed patients are more likely to adhere to protocols; thus, updating them about changes helps them follow the guidelines correctly.

6. **Challenges in Protocol Adaptation**: Despite numerous benefits, adapting protocols faces challenges:

    a. *Data Overload:* With rapidly increasing data from various sources, filtering relevant information can be overwhelming.

    b. *Balancing Consistency and Flexibility:* Adhering strictly to a protocol ensures consistent results but might ignore individual variabilities.

    c. *Cost Implications:* Advanced testing required for personalized adaptations can be expensive.

CHAPTER 3

INTEGRATING PEPTIDES WITH OTHER THERAPIES

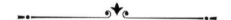

Integrating peptides with other therapies is a new and important area in modern medicine and wellness. When used together with good nutrition and healthy lifestyle changes, peptides can improve overall health. These combinations can make the treatments work better. Peptides can help in many ways, such as boosting the immune system, improving muscle growth, and aiding in recovery from injuries. By using peptides with other treatments, patients can get better results.

For instance, when peptides are used with nutritional plans, it helps the body absorb the nutrients more effectively. Similarly, lifestyle changes like regular exercise and stress management can further enhance the benefits of peptide therapy.

Complementary Nutritional Strategies

When you add peptides to your health routine, eating well is very important. A nutritious diet helps your body make and use peptides better. Without the right nutrients, your body may not be able to produce or use these peptides as effectively, which can impact your overall health and the benefits you get from peptide therapy. Therefore, having a balanced diet full of vitamins, minerals, and other nutrients is essential for making peptide therapy more effective.

1. **Protein-Rich Diet:** Since peptides are made from amino acids, it makes sense to consume sufficient protein. Lean meats, fish, eggs, dairy products, and plant-based proteins like lentils and quinoa are excellent sources. These foods provide the building blocks necessary for peptide synthesis in the body.

2. **Healthy Fats:** Omega-3 fatty acids found in fatty fish, flaxseeds, and walnuts can support cell membrane health which is essential for peptide function. These fats also have anti-inflammatory properties that can enhance the benefits of certain peptides aimed at reducing inflammation.

3. **Micronutrients:** Vitamins and minerals like Vitamin C, Vitamin E, Zinc, and Magnesium play pivotal roles in enzymatic reactions involved in peptide production and utilization:

   a. Vitamin C is crucial for collagen synthesis.
   b. Vitamin E acts as an antioxidant protecting cells.
   c. Zinc assists in protein synthesis.
   d. Magnesium helps with muscle relaxation and enzyme function.

4. **Antioxidant-Rich Foods:** Foods such as berries, leafy greens, nuts, and seeds provide antioxidants that combat oxidative stress. This is particularly beneficial when using peptides for anti-aging or recovery purposes.

By focusing on a balanced diet rich in these nutrients, the efficacy of peptide therapies can be significantly enhanced.

Lifestyle Modifications

Lifestyle choices are fundamental when it comes to integrating peptides effectively into a wellness routine. Certain modifications can amplify the benefits of peptide therapies:

1. **Regular Exercise:** Physical activity stimulates the body's endogenous production of some peptides like growth hormone-releasing peptides (GHRPs). Regular exercise routines that include both aerobic exercises like running or swimming and resistance training like weightlifting can enhance muscle repair, growth, and overall vitality.
2. **Quality Sleep:** Adequate rest is vital for recovery processes where many peptides play a role. Deep sleep phases promote the release of growth hormones which work synergistically with peptide supplements aimed at tissue repair and immune support. Strive for 7-9 hours of sleep per night to optimize this natural process.
3. **Stress Management:** Chronic stress can negatively affect peptide function by disrupting hormonal balance. Techniques such as mindfulness meditation, yoga, deep-breathing exercises, or even hobbies you enjoy can reduce stress levels making the body more responsive to peptide-based interventions.
4. **Hydration:** Staying well-hydrated ensures optimal cellular function including those related to the action of peptides. Aim for at least 8 cups (2 liters) of water per day unless otherwise advised by a healthcare professional.
5. **Avoiding Toxins:** Reduce exposure to environmental toxins like pollutants and cigarette smoke which can hinder peptide effectiveness. Opt for organic produce when possible to avoid pesticides that may disrupt bodily functions tied to peptide activity.
6. **Routine Monitoring:** Regular health check-ups including blood tests can provide insights into how your body is responding to both peptides and other integrated therapies. This allows for timely adjustments ensuring continued efficacy and safety.

Combining with Pharmaceuticals

Combining peptides with pharmaceuticals can offer unique benefits and enhance the therapeutic effects of both types of treatments. Pharmaceuticals are chemically-synthesized compounds designed to target specific pathways or mechanisms within the body to treat diseases. While both have their individual merits, combining them can create a more comprehensive and effective treatment strategy.

One significant advantage of using peptides in conjunction with pharmaceuticals is the complementary action they can provide. For example, a peptide might enhance a specific physiological process while a pharmaceutical targets a different aspect of the same condition. In oncology, combining peptides that boost the immune response with conventional chemotherapy drugs has shown promise. The peptides help to prime the immune system to recognize and attack cancer cells more effectively while chemotherapy works to directly kill those cells.

In treating metabolic disorders like diabetes, combining insulin (a peptide) with other oral hypoglycemic agents can improve glucose control more effectively than either treatment alone. Insulin helps manage blood sugar levels directly, while other medications might increase insulin sensitivity or reduce glucose production by the liver.

When dealing with inflammatory conditions like rheumatoid arthritis or Crohn's disease, peptides that regulate immune system function can be paired with anti-inflammatory pharmaceuticals. This dual approach aims to reduce inflammation more comprehensively by addressing both cytokine activity (through peptides) and broader inflammatory pathways (through drugs).

Combining peptides with pharmaceuticals also involves critical considerations around dosage timing and administration methods. Peptides are generally less stable than traditional drugs and may require special handling or delivery methods, such as injections or advanced drug delivery systems. Ensuring that both therapies reach their target sites at effective concentrations is crucial for achieving the desired outcomes.

It's also important to monitor for potential interactions between peptides and pharmaceuticals, as these could either potentiate or diminish each other's effects. For instance, an increase in enzyme activity from one treatment could lead to a faster degradation of a peptide if not correctly managed. Understanding these dynamics requires thorough research and careful management.

Another consideration is the patient-specific factors like age, genetic profiles, existing health conditions, and current medication regimens. These variables can affect how the body responds to combined therapies. Personalized medicine approaches—tailoring combinations based on individual characteristics—can offer more effective treatments while minimizing adverse effects.

Ethical considerations also arise in developing combined peptide-pharmaceutical therapies. Ensuring access to these cutting-edge treatments for all patient demographics is important. Additionally, long-term studies are necessary to fully understand the safety profiles of new treatment protocols involving combinations of peptides and conventional drugs.

Overall, integrating peptides with pharmaceuticals presents an exciting frontier in medical treatments. This combination allows healthcare providers to exploit the unique strengths of both modalities: leveraging the bioactivity of peptides alongside the potent actions of pharmaceuticals provides an enhanced toolkit for combating various diseases more effectively.

Holistic Health Approaches

Understanding the synergy between peptides and holistic health approaches can significantly enhance your well-being. One compelling reason for combining peptides with holistic health methods is that it addresses not just physical but also emotional and mental aspects of wellness. Holistic health practices stress the connection between mind, body, and spirit. When you use peptides in conjunction with these approaches, you create a multifaceted strategy that bolsters your overall well-being.

Faster Healing and Recovery

Peptides like BPC-157 are renowned for their healing properties. When used alongside holistic techniques such as acupuncture or herbal therapies, the results can be impressive. For example, acupuncture can stimulate the body's own healing processes by improving energy flow or "Qi." When combined with peptide therapy, which actively helps to repair tissues and reduce inflammation, you have a potent toolkit for faster recovery from injuries or surgeries.

METHOD	PEPTIDE	BENEFIT
Acupuncture	BPC-157	Enhanced tissue repair
Herbal Therapy	BPC-157	Reduced inflammation

Enhanced Cognitive Function

Nootropic peptides like Semax are excellent for boosting cognitive function. When combined with mindfulness practices like meditation or yoga, they can produce even more profound effects. Meditation helps by centering the mind and reducing stress, while Semax enhances neuroplasticity, allowing your brain to form new connections more effectively.

Better Sleep Quality

Peptides such as DSIP (Delta Sleep-Inducing Peptide) can aid in achieving better sleep patterns. Pairing this peptide with holistic approaches like aromatherapy or breathwork can help promote deeper and more restorative sleep. Aromatherapy uses essential oils like lavender to create a calming environment conducive to sleep, while DSIP helps regulate sleep cycles at a biochemical level.

Balancing Hormones

Human Growth Hormone (HGH) boosting peptides like CJC-1295 with DAC are useful in regulating hormonal balance. Coupling these with lifestyle changes such as increased physical activity or nutritional adjustments can make the process even more effective. Exercise is known to naturally boost HGH levels, so combining it with CJC-1295 ensures you're maximizing your hormonal health.

Stress Management

Stress is an inevitable part of life but managing it appropriately is crucial for maintaining good health. Peptides such as Epitalon have anti-aging properties and help regulate circadian rhythms which means better stress management and improved mood. Combine Epitalon with practices such as Tai Chi or guided imagery exercises for enhanced stress relief.

Immune Support

Certain peptides bolster immune function effectively when combined with traditional immunity-boosting strategies like sauna sessions or hydration therapy. Thymosin Alpha-1 is one such peptide known for its immune-modulating effects. Sauna sessions elevate your body's core temperature helping you detoxify through sweat; adding Thymosin Alpha-1 magnifies this effect by directly supporting your immune system on a cellular level.

Synergistic Effects

When combining peptides with holistic methods, it's crucial to remember that the sum of these interventions often produces effects greater than their individual parts. This is known as *synergy*. For instance:

PEPTIDE	HOLISTIC PRACTICE	COMBINED EFFECT
Thymosin Beta-4	Massage Therapy	Accelerated muscle recovery
Melanotan II	Sun Exposure & Grounding	Enhanced skin pigmentation and mood

Each person has different needs, so the mix of peptides and holistic methods should be personalized. Consulting with healthcare providers who know both peptides and holistic practices can help create a plan that fits your health goals.

Avoiding Interactions

Integrating peptides with other therapies can be a powerful approach to enhancing health, vitality, and well-being. However, it's crucial to be aware of potential interactions and how to avoid them to ensure safety and effectiveness. When used therapeutically, peptides can offer numerous benefits, including improved immune function, enhanced skin health, and increased muscle mass. Nevertheless, when peptides are combined with other medications or treatments, there is a potential for interactions that could alter their effectiveness or cause adverse effects.

Here are some common interactions that may occur when integrating peptides with other therapies:

1. **Drug-Peptide Interactions**: Peptides can interact with prescription medications in several ways:

   a. *Metabolic Interactions:* Some peptides may affect how drugs are metabolized in the liver. For instance, they could inhibit or induce certain enzymes responsible for drug metabolism.
   b. *Binding Interactions:* Peptides might compete with drugs for binding sites on proteins such as albumin, altering the drugs' distribution and activity.

2. **Supplement-Peptide Interactions**: Nutritional supplements can also interact with peptides:

   a. *Mineral-Binding Interactions:* Certain minerals like calcium or magnesium can bind to peptides and influence their absorption and effectiveness.
   b. *Antioxidant Interactions:* High doses of antioxidants might alter peptide stability or efficacy.

3. **Therapeutic Modality Interactions**: Integration of various therapeutic modalities (like physical therapy or acupuncture) with peptide treatments requires attentiveness:

    a. *Enzymatic Degradation:* Physical activities that increase enzymatic activity might lead to faster degradation of peptides.

    b. *Altered Blood Flow:* Procedures increasing blood flow (like massage) could change peptide distribution and bioavailability.

Strategies to Avoid Interactions

1. **Comprehensive Health Assessment**: Before initiating peptide therapy in conjunction with other treatments, conduct a thorough health assessment. This should include patient history, current medications, supplements intake, and lifestyle habits.

2. **Consultation with Healthcare Providers**: Always consult with healthcare practitioners specializing in peptide therapies who can evaluate potential interactions based on individual patient profiles.

3. **Staggering Administration Times**: Staggering the timing of peptide administration relative to other medications or treatments can minimize interaction risks: For example, taking oral medications at least one hour apart from peptide injections ensures minimal overlap in metabolic pathways.

4. **Monitoring Lab Values**: Regular monitoring of lab values such as liver enzymes and inflammatory markers can help detect early signs of interactions:

LAB TEST	POSSIBLE INTERACTION	RECOMMENDED ACTION
Liver Enzymes	Elevated levels may indicate metabolic interaction	Adjust dosage timings
Inflammatory Markers	Increased levels could point to adverse reactions	Evaluate treatment compatibility

5. **Individualized Dosing Plans**: Develop personalized dosing plans based on the individual's specific needs and responses. Doses of peptides considering factors such as age, weight, genetics, and overall health status.

6. **Effective Communication**: Have open communication channels between patients and healthcare providers. Patients should be encouraged to report any unusual symptoms immediately. Healthcare providers should provide clear instructions regarding the usage of multiple therapies.

CHAPTER 4

TRACKING AND OPTIMIZING RESULTS

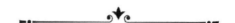

Tracking and optimizing results is essential in any health and wellness plan, including those with peptide treatments. Monitoring your body's response helps you get the most out of your efforts and make necessary adjustments. Keeping detailed records of your daily routines, diet, exercise, and any side effects can show what's working and what needs change. Tracking also helps identify patterns over time, making it easier to see improvements or areas that need more focus.

Optimization ensures that your treatments are tailored for maximum effectiveness. It's not just about adding more peptides or supplements but finding the right balance for you. Understanding how different parts work together can help avoid mistakes that could impact your progress.

Tools for Monitoring Health

With the advancements in technology and medical science, many tools are now available to help individuals monitor their health comprehensively. These tools are important for anyone using peptide protocols. They help you see how well the peptides are working and if they are safe. Tools like blood tests, wearable devices, and health apps can show your body's reaction to peptides. Regular monitoring can catch problems early and make sure you get the best results from your peptide treatment.

Wearable Health Devices

Wearable technology has revolutionized how we monitor our health on a daily basis. Devices like smartwatches and fitness trackers can measure heart rate, sleep patterns, activity levels, and even irregular heartbeats. These gadgets sync with smartphones to provide real-time data at your fingertips.

1. **Heart Rate Monitors:** These are essential for understanding your cardiovascular health. They help you keep track of your heart rate during exercise and rest.
2. **Sleep Trackers:** Quality sleep is vital for recovery and overall health. Sleep trackers provide insights into sleep stages—deep, light, and REM sleep.
3. **Fitness Trackers:** Track steps taken, calories burned, and distance traveled to ensure you are meeting your physical activity goals.
4. **ECG Monitors:** Some advanced wearables include ECG monitors that detect abnormal heart rhythms.

DEVICE	FUNCTION	KEY BENEFITS
Smartwatch	Heart rate monitoring	Real-time updates on cardiovascular health
Fitness Tracker	Physical activity tracking	Motivation to meet daily activity goals
Sleep Tracker	Sleep pattern analysis	Improvement of sleep quality
ECG Monitor	Detection of heart anomalies	Early identification of heart issues

Mobile Health Apps

Mobile health applications have formed an integral part of personalized healthcare management. Many apps allow you to record various health metrics manually or sync with wearable devices.

1. **Diet Tracking Apps:** These apps let you log your daily food intake, offering insights into caloric value, macronutrient breakdowns (proteins, fats, carbohydrates), and nutrient density.
2. **Hydration Reminders:** Proper hydration is essential for every bodily function. Hydration reminder apps calculate your daily water needs based on weight and lifestyle.
3. **Medication Reminders:** Ensure timely intake of peptide doses or other prescribed medications.

Online Health Platforms

Online platforms provide comprehensive tools that centralize all aspects of personal healthcare management.

1. **Health Portals:** Many healthcare providers offer online portals where patients can access their medical records, test results, and scheduling tools.
2. **Telemedicine Services:** Remote consultations with healthcare professionals can save time and make expert advice more accessible.
3. **Online Communities and Support Groups:** Finding a community with similar health goals can provide emotional support and practical advice.

Genetic Testing Kits

Genetic testing can offer unparalleled insights into predisposition toward certain health conditions, helping in the personalization of peptide protocols.

1. **DNA Ancestry Tests:** While primarily designed to trace ancestry, these tests also offer insights into genetic markers associated with specific diseases.

2. **Health Risk Assessment Kits:** These kits assess genetic risk factors for conditions such as heart disease or diabetes.

Biometric Screening

Biometric screenings measure physical characteristics like blood pressure, cholesterol levels, blood glucose levels, etc., to provide a snapshot of your overall health status.

1. **Blood Tests:** Regular blood tests can track changes in important biomarkers such as cholesterol levels or hormone balances affected by peptides.
2. **Urine Analysis Kits:** These kits can offer information about kidney function and metabolic efficiency.
3. **Body Composition Scales:** Advanced scales now measure not just weight but also body fat percentage, muscle mass, and bone density.

Advanced Monitoring Tools

Peptide protocols often require more sophisticated tools for optimal tracking.

1. **Continuous Glucose Monitors (CGMs):** Especially useful for those managing diabetes or concerned with blood sugar levels, CGMs track glucose levels in real-time without the need for frequent finger sticks.
2. **Home Hormone Testing Kits:** These enable users to monitor hormonal imbalances that peptides might address.
3. **Heart Rate Variability (HRV) Monitors:** Measure variations in time between heartbeats as an indicator of stress and overall recovery.

Interpreting Results

Interpreting the results from your peptide protocols is essential for achieving your desired outcomes. It requires careful analysis and understanding of how various peptides interact with your body over time. One of the first steps in interpreting results is recognizing patterns in the data collected during your protocol. This involves looking at various measurable outcomes such as blood markers, body composition changes, and subjective feelings of well-being. Regularly tracking these parameters will help you see trends and make data-driven decisions.

COMMON MEASURABLE OUTCOMES	
PARAMETER	**MEASUREMENT TOOL**
Blood glucose levels	Blood test
Body fat percentage	Body composition scale
Muscle mass	DEXA scan
Energy levels	Subjective assessment

Evaluating Effectiveness

After collecting sufficient data, it's important to evaluate the effectiveness of your peptide protocol. Compare the initial baseline measurements with subsequent data points to determine whether there's improvement, stagnation, or decline.

1. **Improvement:** Consistent positive changes in measurable outcomes suggest that the protocol is effective.
2. **Stagnation:** If there are no significant changes, it might indicate the need for adjustment.
3. **Decline:** Negative trends could mean that the current protocol is not suitable for you.

Correlating Outcomes with Protocol

It's important to correlate specific outcomes with changes made in your peptide regimen. For example, if you notice an increase in muscle mass, identify which peptide or combination of peptides contributed to this change. Example:

1. Peptide A increased energy levels
2. Peptide B + C resulted in decreased body fat percentage

The ability to understand which peptides are producing specific results will help refine your approach.

Monitoring Side Effects

While positive changes are encouraging, monitoring for side effects is equally important. Some peptides may cause adverse reactions such as fatigue, irritability, or gastrointestinal issues. Document any side effects and correlate them with specific peptides and dosages used.

COMMON SIDE EFFECTS AND MANAGEMENT		
SIDE EFFECT	**PEPTIDES INVOLVED**	**MANAGEMENT STRATEGY**
Fatigue	Growth hormone types	Adjust dosage/timing
Gastrointestinal issues	Appetite suppressants	Lower dose/split dosage
Irritability	Fat-burning peptides	Monitor & adjust dosage

Timeframe for Results

Understanding the expected timeframe for seeing results is key to correctly interpreting them. Some peptides may show quick results within weeks, while others may take months. Knowing the typical timeframe helps set realistic expectations and prevents premature discontinuation of a beneficial protocol. Typical timeframes:

1. **Short-term (2-4 weeks):** Initial signs of energy level changes
2. **Mid-term (8-12 weeks):** Observable changes in body composition
3. **Long-term (6+ months):** Significant improvements in overall health markers

Managing Variables

Many factors can influence the effectiveness of a peptide protocol, including diet, exercise, sleep patterns, and stress levels. It's important to manage these variables carefully when interpreting results to ensure that improvements or declines are genuinely due to the peptides. Variables to monitor:

1. **Diet:** Nutrient intake should align with protocol goals.
2. **Exercise:** Consistency and type will impact muscle mass/body fat.
3. **Sleep:** Quality sleep supports recovery and overall health.
4. **Stress:** High stress can counteract benefits from peptide use.

By keeping a close watch on these variables, you can better attribute changes in your measurable outcomes to the peptide protocol rather than other lifestyle factors. For instance, a sudden increase in muscle mass may be more accurately credited to a specific peptide if you know your diet, exercise, sleep, and stress levels have remained constant.

Documenting Results

Keeping detailed records is an invaluable part of interpreting your peptide therapy outcomes. A systematic approach to documentation will enable you to make informed decisions based on factual information rather than anecdotal evidence.

1. **Daily Logs:** Record daily metrics such as energy levels, mood, and any side effects you experience.
2. **Weekly Summaries:** Compile weekly summaries that highlight any significant changes in measurable outcomes like weight, body composition, and blood markers.
3. **Monthly Reviews:** Monthly reviews help in identifying long-term trends by comparing data over extended periods.

When to Modify Protocols

Achieving the desired outcomes using peptide protocols involves careful planning and ongoing adjustments. Peptide protocols are not a one-size-fits-all solution. Several factors determine when modifications are necessary:

1. **Non-Responsiveness:** If you notice that the anticipated results are not materializing within the expected timeframe, it might be time to reassess the protocol. This could involve changing the dosage, switching peptides, or combining different peptides.
2. **Plateau Effect:** Often in peptide therapy, users experience initial positive changes that may hit a plateau. If progress stalls despite adherence to the regimen, a tweak may help to push past this plateau.
3. **Side Effects:** Users may encounter side effects such as headaches, fatigue, or skin reactions. If side effects occur, modifying the dose or frequency can mitigate these reactions while still achieving desired outcomes.
4. **Individual Goals:** Personal goals may evolve over time. For instance, someone initially looking for energy boosts might later focus on muscle growth or cognitive enhancements. Such shifting objectives necessitate protocol adjustments.

Here's a simple table highlighting when to consider modifying protocols:

Condition	Indicative Action
Non-Responsiveness	Reassess dosage or peptide combination
Plateau Effect	Adjust regimen to break stagnation
Side Effects	Modify dose/frequency to reduce adverse effects
Change in Goals	Tailor peptides to align with revised objectives

Long-Term Considerations

Long-term use of peptide therapies brings specific considerations. These factors ensure sustained benefits without compromising overall health:

1. **Rotational Scheduling:** To prevent desensitization or reduced efficacy, implementing rotational schedules (cycling different peptides) can prove beneficial. Continuous use of the same peptide might decrease its effectiveness over time.
2. **Monitoring Biomarkers:** Regular health check-ups focusing on biomarkers relevant to your protocol should guide long-term usage strategies. Metrics such as hormone levels, liver functions, and inflammation markers help optimize ongoing treatments.
3. **Gradual Dosing:** Starting with lower doses and gradually increasing can minimize potential side effects and allow your body to adjust smoothly. Over time, this helps in finding the optimal balance for effectiveness and tolerability.
4. **Sustainable Practices:** Incorporating peptides into a broader wellness strategy is crucial. Complement peptides with good nutrition, exercise, and adequate sleep to enhance their effects and contribute to overall well-being.
5. **Periodic Reviews:** Routine consultations with a healthcare provider experienced in peptide therapy ensure the protocol remains relevant to your evolving needs and health status.

Success Metrics

Success metrics are vital because they offer a systemic way to determine if peptide protocols are working effectively. By monitoring these metrics, you can fine-tune your approach, ensuring you're continually making progress toward your wellness goals. Key areas to focus on include physical health, mental well-being, and overall vitality.

Physical Health Metrics

1. **Body Composition:** Measuring body fat and muscle mass can provide insights into how peptides affect your physique. Tools like DEXA scans, bioelectrical impedance analysis (BIA), and skinfold calipers are effective methods.

Metric	Optimal Range
Body Fat	Men: 10-20%, Women: 20-30%
Muscle Mass	Varied based on age/gender

2. **Blood Markers:** Regular blood tests can reveal critical information about your internal health. Important markers include:

   a. *Hormone Levels:* Testosterone, estrogen, insulin growth factor (IGF-1)
   b. *Metabolic Markers:* Blood glucose levels, lipid profile
   c. *Inflammatory Markers:* C-reactive protein (CRP), cytokines

3. **Vital Signs:** Basic vitals provide foundational health information.

   a. *Blood Pressure:* Aim for 120/80 mmHg
   b. *Heart Rate:* Resting heart rate should be between 60-100 bpm
   c. *Respiratory Rate:* Normal rate is 12-20 breaths per minute

Mental Well-being Metrics

1. **Cognitive Function Tests:** Tools like the Montreal Cognitive Assessment (MoCA) or Mini-Mental State Examination (MMSE) can help monitor cognitive changes.
2. **Mood Assessments:** Standard questionnaires such as the Beck Depression Inventory (BDI) or Generalized Anxiety Disorder scale (GAD-7) can be useful.
3. **Sleep Quality:** Tracking sleep patterns using devices such as smart watches or apps helps assess sleep duration and quality which are critical for brain function and overall health.

Vitality Metrics

1. **Energy Levels:** Keeping a daily log of your energy levels can offer insights.
2. **Exercise Performance:** Track improvements in your physical activities such as running times, weights lifted, or yoga progressions.
3. **Quality of Life Scores:** Surveys like the WHOQOL-BREF (World Health Organization Quality of Life Questionnaire) give a holistic snapshot of well-being.

While these metrics provide a general framework, it is crucial to tailor them to personal needs and goals. Not everyone's optimal ranges will look the same due to factors like age, sex, genetic predisposition, and lifestyle choices.

Continual assessment allows for adjustments in peptide dosages or types being used. For instance, if muscle mass gain is slower than desired despite everything else being optimal, your protocol might require a different peptide or adjusted dosage.

CHAPTER 5

ADVANCED APPLICATIONS

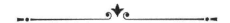

Scientific advancements in peptide research have paved the way for groundbreaking applications that impact various aspects of health and well-being. These advanced applications are crucial because they offer novel solutions to complex medical challenges and open up new frontiers in therapeutic approaches. By exploring these cutting-edge methods, healthcare professionals can develop more targeted treatments with fewer side effects, ultimately improving patient outcomes.

Furthermore, understanding and leveraging these advances can lead to personalized medicine—where treatments are tailored to meet individual needs based on genetic profiles. This level of precision in healthcare represents a significant leap from the traditional one-size-fits-all approach, ensuring more effective and efficient interventions. Additionally, advanced peptide applications also have the potential to enhance longevity by addressing age-related conditions at their molecular roots.

Research Frontiers

Peptide therapy is at the forefront of medical research, opening new possibilities for treating complex health issues. Scientists are exploring how peptides can influence various biological processes, offering promising results in disease treatment and prevention.

One primary area of research is cancer treatment. Traditional therapies like chemotherapy and radiation can have significant side effects and may not be effective for all cancer types. Peptides offer a targeted approach by binding specifically to cancer cells, minimizing damage to healthy tissues. Researchers are developing peptide-based drugs that can penetrate tumor cells and deliver cytotoxic agents precisely where they are needed, improving treatment efficacy and reducing side effects.

Another exciting frontier is neurodegenerative diseases like Alzheimer's and Parkinson's. These conditions have limited treatment options and devastating impacts on patients' lives. Peptides are being studied for their ability to cross the blood-brain barrier—an obstacle that prevents many drugs from reaching the brain. Peptides designed to target specific receptors or pathways in the brain could potentially slow down or even reverse the progression of these diseases.

Moreover, peptides are being researched for their roles in metabolic disorders such as diabetes and obesity. Certain peptides can mimic hormones that regulate appetite, glucose metabolism, and insulin sensitivity. By modulating these biological processes, peptide therapies could offer new solutions for managing weight and blood sugar levels more effectively than current medications.

Additionally, cardiovascular health is benefiting from peptide research. Peptides that promote vasodilation—widening of blood vessels—can improve circulation and reduce blood pressure. Other peptides are being developed to repair damaged heart tissue following a heart attack, which could dramatically improve recovery outcomes for patients.

Experimental Peptides

The development of experimental peptides is pushing the boundaries of what modern medicine can achieve. Laboratories worldwide are synthesizing new peptides and testing their effects in preclinical studies. One such example is BPC-157 (Body Protection Compound 157). This peptide is derived from a protein found in human gastric juice. Studies suggest BPC-157 has powerful regenerative properties, aiding in muscle healing, tendon repair, and even intestinal health.

Another promising experimental peptide is Thymosin Beta-4 (TB-500). Found naturally in high concentrations in blood platelets, TB-500 promotes cell migration and wound healing. Researchers are investigating its potential for treating chronic injuries and enhancing recovery from surgeries.

Epitalon is another intriguing peptide undergoing research for its anti-aging properties. It works by regulating the production of telomerase, an enzyme crucial for maintaining telomere length at the ends of chromosomes. Shortened telomeres are associated with aging and various diseases; by promoting telomere elongation, Epitalon could potentially extend lifespan and delay age-related conditions.

In muscle growth and athletic performance enhancement, peptides like Ipamorelin stand out due to their ability to stimulate growth hormone release without many adverse effects linked to synthetic growth hormones. This property makes them attractive for treating growth hormone deficiencies or enhancing physical performance legally within regulatory guidelines.

Peptides influencing cognitive functions are also under examination. Cerebrolysin—a mix of neuropeptides—has shown promise in enhancing memory, protecting neurons from damage, and improving outcomes after strokes or traumatic brain injuries.

While these experimental peptides show significant promise, it's important to emphasize that many remain under study and are not yet available as approved treatments through conventional medical channels. The safety profiles, long-term effects, and broader applications require thorough investigation through clinical trials before they can be widely recommended.

Peptide Stacks

Peptide stacking refers to the strategic use of multiple peptides in conjunction, aimed at maximizing health benefits. When used alone, peptides can be effective in targeting specific physiological processes, but when combined in carefully considered stacks, the results can be far more profound. Much like combining vitamins for improved nutrition, peptide stacks can augment each other's effects.

1. **Synergistic Effects**: The primary advantage of peptide stacks is their synergistic effect. For instance, using a Growth Hormone Releasing Peptide (GHRP) alongside a Growth Hormone Releasing Hormone (GHRH) can lead to a more substantial increase in growth hormone levels than using either alone. This kind of synergy allows for optimized therapeutic outcomes while minimizing doses and potential side effects.

2. **Customized Protocols**: Everyone's physiology is unique, and one-size-fits-all solutions often fall short. By customizing peptide stacks tailored to individual needs—whether it's for anti-aging, muscle growth, or cognitive function—practitioners can address specific health goals more effectively. An example of a commonly used stack for muscle growth might include CJC-1295 (a GHRH) and Ipamorelin (a GHRP). Another stack could involve BPC-157 and TB-500 for tissue repair and inflammation reduction.

3. **Enhanced Bioavailability**: The effectiveness of peptides can sometimes be limited by their bioavailability; that is, how well they are absorbed and utilized by the body. Certain peptides, when stacked together, can improve each other's bioavailability. For example, combining a peptide with a carrier protein might improve its stability and absorption rate.

4. **Diverse Applications**: Depending on the goal, peptide stacks have various applications:

   a. *Anti-Aging:* A typical anti-aging stack could include Epitalon and thymosin alpha-1 to improve immune function along with promoting longevity.
   b. *Fat Loss:* Combining AOD9604 with CJC-1295/Ipamorelin might enhance fat metabolism while preserving lean muscle mass.
   c. *Cognitive Enhancement:* Peptides like Dihexa paired with Cerebrolysin can potentially boost cognitive performance and neural health.

Genetic Considerations

Understanding individual genetic make-up can drastically improve the outcomes of peptide protocols. Genetic considerations involve tailoring peptide use to align with one's genetic predispositions.

1. **Personalized Medicine Approaches:** By analyzing an individual's genome, specific peptides can be recommended to mitigate genetic risks or enhance particular strengths. For example, someone genetically predisposed to osteoporosis might benefit more from peptides like Forteo or Teriparatide that promote bone density.

2. **Epigenetics:** Epigenetic modifications determine how genes are expressed without changing the DNA sequence. Peptides like Epitalon have been found to induce favorable epigenetic changes that correlate with longevity markers across multiple studies.

3. **Polymorphisms Affecting Peptide Efficacy:** Polymorphisms are variations in DNA sequences that can affect how well certain peptides work. The Val66Met polymorphism in the BDNF gene affects brain-derived neurotrophic factor

levels; individuals with this variant may respond differently to peptides promoting cognitive enhancement such as Cerebrolysin.

4. **Nutrigenomics:** This is the study of food's effect on gene expression related to health and disease prevention. Peptides designed to optimize metabolism can be more effective when complementing a diet tailored to one's genetic makeup. For instance, those with a tendency towards poor lipid metabolism could see pronounced benefits from combining metabolic peptides with a low-fat diet.

Future of Peptide Therapies

The future of peptide therapies holds immense promise for medical and health practices. One of the exciting developments in peptide therapy is its application in chronic disease management. For instance, peptides have shown promise in treating diabetes by acting on specific receptors to regulate blood sugar levels. This could potentially reduce the dependence on insulin injections for many patients. Additionally, peptides might offer solutions for heart diseases by promoting tissue repair and reducing inflammation.

Cancer treatment is another area where peptide therapies are making significant strides. Traditional cancer treatments like chemotherapy and radiation can have severe side effects and often damage healthy tissues. Peptides offer a targeted approach to treatment, aiming to deliver drugs directly to cancer cells without affecting normal cells. This specificity reduces side effects and improves the efficacy of treatments.

Peptide therapies also hold potential in combating neurodegenerative diseases such as Alzheimer's and Parkinson's. Research has shown that certain peptides can cross the blood-brain barrier, allowing direct intervention in the brain. These peptides might help in breaking down abnormal protein aggregates that are characteristic of these diseases or even promote neural regeneration.

In the field of infectious diseases, peptide-based vaccines and anti-viral treatments are being intensively studied. Peptide vaccines could offer a way to stimulate the immune system more effectively by mimicking parts of pathogens that the body can easily recognize and respond to. This approach is not only seen in combating existing diseases but also holds promise for rapidly developing vaccines against emerging threats.

Moreover, peptide therapies are gaining momentum in anti-aging and cosmetic applications. Collagen peptides, for example, are widely used to promote skin health by improving moisture retention and elasticity. The role of peptides in muscle growth and fat loss is also being explored extensively, showing benefits for physical fitness and body composition.

Peptide research is not just limited to human medicine; veterinary science is also benefiting from these advances. Pets with chronic conditions or age-related issues could see improvements through peptide treatments aimed at reducing inflammation or enhancing immunity.

As we look towards the future, one crucial aspect will be the delivery systems of these therapies. Ensuring that peptides reach their target sites efficiently without degradation will be a significant focus area. Innovations such as nanotechnology-enhanced delivery systems and novel formulations are expected to enhance the stability and bioavailability of peptide drugs.

BOOK 3

PEPTIDE HEALTH AND HEALING

CHAPTER 1

HEALING WITH PEPTIDES

Peptides are powerful allies in the body's healing processes. One of the most compelling reasons to explore healing with peptides is their potential to promote faster and more effective recovery from various injuries and ailments. Peptides have shown significant promise in reducing inflammation, which is a root cause of many chronic conditions. Inflammation can lead to prolonged pain, swelling, and discomfort, hampering everyday activities and overall well-being. By using peptides to manage and reduce inflammation, individuals can experience quicker relief and improved quality of life.

Furthermore, peptides are integral to tissue repair and regeneration. When tissues are damaged due to injury or surgery, peptides facilitate the formation of new cells and tissues, expediting the healing process. This can be particularly beneficial for athletes or anyone undergoing rehabilitation after an injury.

As we age, our bodies naturally undergo wear and tear. Peptides offer a way to potentially slow down this aging process by supporting cellular health and function. Their anti-aging effects can contribute to longer-lasting vitality and youthfulness. Lastly, peptides have been found to improve metabolic health by regulating insulin levels and supporting weight management. Improved metabolism not only aids in maintaining a healthy weight but also reduces the risk of conditions like diabetes and cardiovascular disease.

Anti-Inflammatory Effects

Inflammation is a key part of our body's immune response, but when it becomes chronic, it can lead to various diseases. Peptides have emerged as powerful agents with anti-inflammatory properties, showing great promise in treating a variety of conditions linked to inflammation. One significant way peptides exert their anti-inflammatory effects is by blocking the action of inflammatory cytokines, which are proteins that signal cells to initiate an inflammatory response.

Key Peptides with Anti-Inflammatory Effects

1. **BPC-157:** BPC-157 is a synthetic peptide derived from a protein found in the stomach. It has been shown to have profound anti-inflammatory effects, particularly in tissues like muscles, tendons, and the gut. BPC-157 works by modulating several growth factors and promoting angiogenesis (the formation of new blood vessels), which aids in tissue repair and reduces inflammation.
2. **Thymosin Beta-4 (TB-500):** TB-500 is another powerful peptide known for its ability to reduce inflammation and promote healing. It plays a role in regulating the actin cytoskeleton, which is essential for cell movement and regeneration. By doing so, TB-500 helps reduce inflammatory responses, promoting faster recovery from injuries and decreasing the persistence of chronic inflammatory states.
3. **Melanotan II:** Primarily known for its skin tanning benefits, Melanotan II also exhibits anti-inflammatory properties. It works by activating melanocortin receptors, which participate in immune system regulation and inflammation control.
4. **Epithalon:** Epithalon is a tetrapeptide with notable anti-aging properties through its regulation of telomerase activity. However, it also possesses significant anti-inflammatory effects by modulating cytokine production and reducing oxidative stress within cells.

Mechanisms of Action

The following table outlines some key mechanisms through which peptides exert their anti-inflammatory effects:

PEPTIDE	MECHANISM	RESULTS
BPC-157	Modulation of growth factors; angiogenesis	Reduced tissue inflammation
TB-500	Regulation of actin cytoskeleton	Enhanced healing; reduced swelling
Melanotan II	Activation of melanocortin receptors	Improved immune response
Epithalon	Modulation of cytokine production; antioxidation	Decreased oxidative stress

How Peptides Combat Inflammation

1. **Inhibition of Pro-inflammatory Cytokines:** Peptides can reduce the production of cytokines which are small proteins important in cell signaling. Cytokines like TNF-alpha and IL-6 are often elevated in chronic inflammation. Specific peptides have been identified that inhibit these cytokines, thereby reducing inflammation.
2. **Antioxidant Activity:** Some peptides exhibit antioxidant properties that neutralize free radicals in the body. This is essential because free radicals can fuel the inflammatory process.
3. **Immune Modulation:** Peptides can balance immune system activity by promoting anti-inflammatory pathways while dampening the pro-inflammatory ones, ensuring a balanced immune response.

Applications in Enhancing Longevity

Chronic inflammation is connected with aging and age-related diseases. By targeting the inflammatory pathways, peptides can significantly contribute to healthy aging:

1. **Arthritis Management:** People suffering from rheumatoid arthritis or osteoarthritis can benefit immensely from peptides like BPC-157 which aid in reducing joint pain and promoting cartilage repair.
2. **Heart Health:** Chronic inflammation is a major risk factor for heart disease. Anti-inflammatory peptides could offer a novel approach for managing cardiovascular health by mitigating inflammation-induced damage.
3. **Neuroprotection:** Emerging evidence suggests that inflammation plays a key role in neurodegenerative diseases like Alzheimer's and Parkinson's. Certain peptides have shown potential in protecting neuronal cells from inflammatory damage.

Tissue Repair and Regeneration

Tissue repair and regeneration are natural processes that the body uses to heal and re-grow damaged tissue. These processes are crucial for maintaining the overall health and functionality of an organism. This section explores the mechanisms underlying tissue repair and regeneration, focusing on their significance, types of tissue involved, and factors that influence these processes.

There are two main types of tissue repair: regeneration and fibrosis.

1. **Regeneration:** This process involves the replacement of damaged or dead cells with identical new ones. It relies on the body's ability to proliferate specific cell types to restore tissue function completely.
2. **Fibrosis:** This type of repair happens when the damaged tissue is replaced with scar tissue, which is predominantly made up of collagen. While scar tissue helps maintain structural integrity, it does not restore the original functionality of the organ or tissue.

Phases of Tissue Repair

Tissue repair generally involves four phases:

1. Hemostasis

- ➤ This is the immediate response after tissue injury.
- ➤ Blood vessels constrict to reduce bleeding.
- ➤ Platelets aggregate to form a clot.

2. Inflammation

- ➤ Cells release chemicals that initiate inflammation.
- ➤ Inflammatory cells migrate to the site of injury.
- ➤ These cells clean up debris and bacteria.

3. **Proliferation**

- ➤ New tissue forms as fibroblasts produce collagen and extracellular matrix (ECM).
- ➤ Angiogenesis occurs, creating new blood vessels.
- ➤ Epithelial cells proliferate and cover the wound.

4. **Remodeling**

- ➤ The wound contracts as collagen fibers are realigned.
- ➤ Scar tissue becomes stronger but less flexible than original tissue.

Factors Influencing Tissue Repair and Regeneration

Several factors can affect how well tissues repair themselves:

1. **Age**: Younger individuals usually have a higher regenerative capacity compared to older individuals.

2. **Nutrition**: Adequate levels of proteins, vitamins (especially A, C, and E), and minerals are necessary for optimal tissue repair.

3. **Blood Supply**: Tissues with a good blood supply tend to heal faster due to better delivery of oxygen and nutrients.

4. **Health Conditions**: Chronic illnesses like diabetes can slow down the process of healing.

5. **Peptides:** Peptides can significantly enhance tissue repair by stimulating cellular activities essential for regeneration.

Peptides promote efficient tissue repair and regeneration. They can be engineered or derived naturally based on amino acid sequences that mimic naturally occurring peptides involved in body regulation.

PEPTIDE	MECHANISM	RESULTS
BPC-157	Accelerates angiogenesis (formation of new blood vessels)	Faster wound healing
Thymosin Beta-4	Promotes cell migration to injury site	Improved nerve repair; reduces scar formation
GHK-Cu	Modulates genes related to healing	Anti-inflammatory; increases collagen production

These peptides can aid in reducing inflammation, accelerating cell migration to wounds, promoting new blood vessel formation, and increasing collagen deposition—all crucial steps in effective tissue repair.

Neuroprotective Properties

Neurons are the building blocks of our nervous system and are responsible for processing and transmitting information. Maintaining their health is crucial for cognitive function, motor skills, and emotional well-being. Neurodegenerative diseases such as Alzheimer's, Parkinson's, and Multiple Sclerosis (MS) are primarily characterized by the progressive loss of neuron function. Factors contributing to neuron damage include oxidative stress, inflammation, abnormal protein aggregation, and mitochondrial dysfunction. In recent years, specific peptides have been identified with properties that protect neurons from damage and support their function. Let's explore some of these key peptides.

1. **BPC-157 (Body Protection Compound-157):** BPC-157 is known for its regenerative properties. It helps reduce inflammation in neural tissues and promotes healing by enhancing blood flow to injured areas. Research has indicated significant improvement in recovery from traumatic brain injuries when treated with BPC-157.

2. **Cerebrolysin:** This peptide mixture contains several neurotrophic factors. It supports neurogenesis (the growth of new neurons) and protects existing neurons from apoptosis (programmed cell death). Widely used in Europe for treating stroke and traumatic brain injuries; it has shown benefits in cognitive functions.

3. **Selank:** Selank is derived from tuftsin, which is a natural immunomodulatory peptide. It reduces anxiety and has anti-inflammatory effects on the nervous system. Commonly used for its anxiolytic effects without causing sedation.

4. **Semax:** Semax is a synthetic analog of the ACTH fragment. It enhances cognitive functions and protects against oxidative stress. Applied in Russia for treating ischemic stroke and cognitive disorders.

5. **Thymosin Beta-4 (TB-500):** TB-500 is a potent anti-inflammatory agent. It promotes regeneration by aiding in cell migration, maturation, and differentiation. Used experimentally to aid recovery from nervous system traumas.

PEPTIDE	MECHANISM	CLINICAL APPLICATIONS
BPC-157	Anti- inflammatory, healing promotion	Traumatic brain injury
Cerebrolysin	Supports neurogenesis	Stroke recovery
Selank	Reduces anxiety	Anxiety management
Semax	Enhances cognition	Cognitive enhancement post-stroke
Thymosin Beta-4	Cell regeneration	Nervous system trauma recovery

Mechanisms Underlying Neuroprotection

Several mechanisms have been proposed for how these peptides exert their neuroprotective effects:

1. **Reduction of Oxidative Stress:** Oxidative stress occurs when there is an imbalance between free radicals and antioxidants in the body. Free radicals can damage neurons, leading to their dysfunction or death. Neuroprotective peptides often help balance this by either reducing the production of free radicals or by enhancing the action of antioxidants in neural tissues. For example, Semax has been shown to decrease oxidative stress markers, thus protecting neurons from damage.

2. **Anti-inflammatory Effects:** Inflammation in the nervous system can result from injuries, infections, or chronic diseases and can lead to neuron damage. Peptides like BPC-157 and Thymosin Beta-4 have potent anti-inflammatory effects that help reduce this inflammation and protect neurons. These peptides reduce the production of inflammatory cytokines and inhibit pathways that lead to chronic inflammation.

3. **Promotion of Neurogenesis:** Neurogenesis refers to the process by which new neurons are formed in the brain. Cerebrolysin promotes neurogenesis by supporting the growth of new neurons and the survival of existing ones. It contains several growth factors that stimulate neuronal stem cells, encouraging them to differentiate into mature neurons.

4. **Inhibition of Apoptosis:** Apoptosis is a form of programmed cell death that is essential for normal development but can be harmful when uncontrolled. Peptides like Cerebrolysin help to inhibit apoptosis in neurons, ensuring their survival especially under stressful conditions such as oxygen deprivation (ischemia) during a stroke.

5. **Enhancement of Blood Flow:** Adequate blood flow is essential for delivering oxygen and nutrients to brain tissues. BPC-157 improves blood circulation and aids in healing processes following neural injuries by promoting angiogenesis—the formation of new blood vessels—thereby ensuring neurons receive sufficient oxygen and nutrients for repair.

Anti-Aging Effects

As we age, the pursuit of a longer, more vibrant life becomes a central focus. Various factors contribute to the aging process, including genetics, lifestyle choices, and environmental influences. However, recent research has identified peptides as a promising avenue for combating the signs of aging and enhancing overall longevity and vitality. Peptides exert their anti-aging effects through several mechanisms:

1. **Collagen Stimulation:** Collagen is a protein found in skin, hair, and connective tissues. As we age, collagen production declines, leading to wrinkles and sagging skin. Certain peptides can stimulate collagen synthesis, thereby improving skin elasticity and firmness.
2. **Antioxidant Properties:** Oxidative stress damages cells and accelerates aging. Peptides with antioxidant properties can neutralize free radicals, reducing cellular damage and promoting longevity.
3. **Cellular Repair:** Some peptides enhance the body's ability to repair damaged cells and tissues. This is crucial for maintaining optimal function in organs like the heart and brain as we age.
4. **Hormonal Balance:** Peptides can modulate hormone levels, which often decline with age. For instance, growth hormone-releasing peptides stimulate the release of growth hormones, promoting muscle mass maintenance and fat metabolism.

Specific Peptides for Anti-Aging

Several specific peptides have been identified for their potential anti-aging benefits:

1. **GHK-Cu (Copper Peptide):** Works by repairing tissue damage and stimulating collagen production.
2. **Epitalon:** This peptide regulates telomerase activity, an enzyme that maintains telomere length in DNA strands. Longer telomeres are associated with increased lifespan.
3. **Thymosin Beta-4:** Aids in tissue regeneration and reduces inflammation.

The practical benefits of anti-aging peptides are supported by both clinical studies and anecdotal evidence:

1. **Skin Aging:** Topical application of GHK-Cu has shown significant improvements in skin appearance by reducing fine lines, increasing skin thickness, and enhancing overall skin tone.

2. **Physical Vitality:** In studies involving elderly populations, epitalon administration led to improvements in physical functioning and reduced occurrences of age-related diseases.
3. **Cognitive Health:** Peptides like Cerebrolysin have been linked to enhanced cognitive function and neuroprotection in aging individuals.

PEPTIDE	MECHANISM	APPLICATION
GHK-Cu	Skin rejuvenation	Topical
Epitalon	Telomere lengthening	Injection
Thymosin Beta-4	Tissue repair	Injection
Growth Hormone-Releasing Peptides (GHRPs)	Hormone balance	Injection
Cerebrolysin	Cognitive enhancement	Injection

While peptides offer promising anti-aging benefits, it's essential to use them under professional guidance. The quality of peptide products varies widely, so sourcing from reputable suppliers is crucial for safety and effectiveness.

Metabolic Health Improvements

One area where peptides have shown significant promise is in improving metabolic health. Metabolic health pertains to how well our bodies generate and use energy, and it encompasses processes like glucose regulation, fat metabolism, and energy expenditure. Poor metabolic health can lead to conditions such as obesity, diabetes, and cardiovascular diseases. Some peptides can influence metabolic processes directly by mimicking or stimulating the activity of certain hormones or enzymes.

1. **GLP-1 (Glucagon-Like Peptide-1):** One of the most researched peptides in the context of metabolic health is Glucagon-Like Peptide-1 (GLP-1). This peptide is naturally produced in the gut in response to food intake. GLP-1 enhances insulin secretion from the pancreas, which helps lower blood glucose levels. By doing so, it plays a crucial role in blood sugar regulation.

Furthermore, GLP-1 also slows down gastric emptying, which promotes a feeling of fullness and aids in weight management. Drugs that mimic GLP-1 (GLP-1 agonists) are currently being used to treat type 2 diabetes and obesity effectively.

2. **CJC-1295:** CJC-1295 is another peptide associated with improvements in metabolic health. It stimulates the release of growth hormone from the pituitary gland. Growth hormone has several functions, including increasing muscle mass and decreasing body fat. By promoting better muscle-to-fat ratio, CJC-1295 supports improved metabolic rates and greater energy expenditure.

Additionally, growth hormone can influence lipid metabolism by encouraging the body to use fat as a primary energy source rather than carbohydrates. This shift can significantly assist individuals looking to reduce fat mass and improve overall body composition.

3. **AOD9604:** AOD9604 is a fragment of human growth hormone that specifically targets fat reduction without influencing blood sugar or producing unwanted effects typical with whole growth hormone administration. Studies

have suggested that AOD9604 exerts its actions by mimicking the way natural growth hormone regulates fat metabolism.

This peptide enhances lipolysis—the breakdown of fats—and inhibits lipogenesis—the creation of new fat cells—thereby supporting weight loss efforts and improved metabolic function without disturbing other hormonal axes.

4. **MOTS-c**: MOTS-c is a mitochondrial-derived peptide that has drawn attention due to its role in promoting metabolic flexibility—the ability of cells to switch between burning different types of fuel sources like glucose and fatty acids efficiently. This adaptability is crucial for maintaining good metabolic health.

Research indicates that MOTS-c can improve insulin sensitivity and increase skeletal muscle uptake of glucose. These effects support better glycemic control and enhanced energy levels, making MOTS-c a promising candidate for managing metabolic disorders such as diabetes.

CHAPTER 2

PEPTIDES AND DISEASE MANAGEMENT

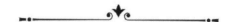

Peptides are important in managing diseases because they target specific areas in the body and have fewer side effects than traditional treatments. They can bind to particular receptors, which helps them work exactly where needed and reduces the risk of affecting unintended parts of the body. This precision makes peptides a popular choice for various treatments. They are used in cancer therapy and for controlling chronic diseases like diabetes.

Peptides are significantly advancing medical treatments and improving how we manage many health conditions. Let's look into some important areas where peptides are making significant progress in disease management.

Peptides in Cancer Therapy

One promising application of peptides in cancer therapy is the development of peptide-based vaccines. Unlike traditional vaccines that prevent infectious diseases, cancer vaccines aim to treat existing tumors by stimulating the body's immune response to target and destroy cancer cells. Scientists identify specific antigens present on tumor cells and design peptides that mimic these antigens. When introduced into the body, these synthetic peptides train the immune system to recognize and attack cancer cells bearing those antigens.

Another critical development in peptide-related cancer therapies involves checkpoint inhibitors. The immune system utilizes checkpoints—proteins on immune cells that need to be activated (or inactivated) to start an immune response. Some cancers exploit these checkpoints to avoid being attacked by the immune system. Peptides can be engineered to inhibit these checkpoints, thereby boosting the body's ability to attack cancer cells.

Peptide-drug conjugates (PDCs) represent a novel strategy for delivering therapeutic agents directly to cancer cells while sparing healthy tissue. PDCs are composed of a peptide linked to a potent anti-cancer drug. The peptide component targets specific receptors on cancer cells, ensuring that the drug is delivered precisely where it's needed most. This method increases the effectiveness of the drug and reduces side effects commonly associated with chemotherapy.

Tumors require a blood supply to grow and spread, a process known as angiogenesis. Certain peptides can inhibit angiogenesis by blocking the signals tumors send out to initiate blood vessel growth. By preventing new blood vessel formation, these peptides essentially starve the tumor, limiting its growth and ability to metastasize.

Many peptide-based therapies are currently undergoing clinical trials, showing promise in treating various types of cancers including melanoma, breast cancer, and prostate cancer. For instance, there have been notable advancements in "theranostic" peptides, designed for both therapy and diagnostics.

APPLICATION	MECHANISM	BENEFITS	EXAMPLES
Cancer Vaccines	Stimulate immune response	Targeted immunity	NY-ESO-1 Peptide Vaccine
Checkpoint Inhibitors	Block immune checkpoints	Boosts body's natural defenses	Pembrolizumab
Peptide-Drug Conjugates	Direct delivery of drugs	Higher effectiveness, reduced side effects	Zoptarelin Doxorubicin
Angiogenesis Inhibitors	Block blood vessel formation	Starves tumor cells	Bevacizumab (Avastin)

The future for peptides in cancer therapy looks incredibly promising as researchers continue to explore new ways to harness their potential. Advances in biotechnology and molecular biology will further enhance our understanding of how peptides can be used more effectively. Areas like personalized medicine—where treatments are tailored specifically based on an individual's genetic makeup—are likely to benefit significantly from peptide research.

Peptides in Cardiovascular Health

Peptides are small proteins that help protect and improve heart and blood vessel functions. They are important in cardiovascular health because they can lower blood pressure, reduce inflammation, and help repair damaged tissues. These benefits can help prevent heart diseases and improve overall heart health. Peptides are currently being studied for their potential as treatments for various heart conditions including heart attack recovery and high blood pressure. Understanding the role of peptides in keeping the cardiovascular system healthy is crucial, as this knowledge could lead to new, more effective therapies for heart diseases.

One of the key areas where peptides show promise is in the regulation of blood pressure. Angiotensin-converting enzyme (ACE) inhibitors are well-known medications used to treat high blood pressure. Interestingly, certain peptides can inhibit ACE, thereby preventing the conversion of angiotensin I to the more potent vasoconstrictor angiotensin II. This helps to relax blood vessels and lower blood pressure. Peptides like Valyl-Prolyl-Proline (VPP) and Isoleucyl-Prolyl-Proline (IPP) are examples of naturally occurring ACE inhibitors found in dairy products.

High cholesterol levels are a risk factor for cardiovascular diseases. Peptides have been found to help in managing cholesterol levels by interfering with its absorption in the intestines or by directly affecting cholesterol metabolism. Soy peptides, for instance, have been shown to lower LDL (bad) cholesterol while having negligible effects on HDL (good) cholesterol. This makes them a useful tool in managing dyslipidemia.

Inflammation is important in the development of atherosclerosis, which is the hardening or narrowing of the arteries due to plaque buildup. Peptides like Melanotan-II have shown anti-inflammatory properties that could help reduce the risk of atherosclerosis. By decreasing inflammation, these peptides can potentially slow down or even prevent the progression of cardiovascular diseases.

Oxidative stress is another contributing factor to cardiovascular diseases. Reactive oxygen species can damage cells and tissues, leading to conditions such as atherosclerosis and heart failure. Some peptides possess antioxidant properties that neutralize these reactive molecules, thereby protecting cardiovascular tissues. Glutathione is one such peptide that acts as a powerful antioxidant and plays a crucial role in maintaining cardiovascular health.

Your body has an incredible ability to repair itself, and peptides play a significant role in this process, particularly concerning cardiovascular tissues. Thymosin Beta-4 is a peptide that promotes tissue repair and regeneration. It aids in angiogenesis (formation of new blood vessels) and can even reduce scar tissue formation after heart injuries like myocardial infarction.

Peptides also play roles in directly enhancing cardiac function. For example, B-type Natriuretic Peptide (BNP) helps regulate blood pressure and fluid balance through natriuresis (excretion of sodium through urine). Elevated levels of BNP are often associated with heart failure; however, synthetic analogs have been developed for therapeutic purposes.

PEPTIDE	MECHANISM	Potential Benefits
VPP & IPP	ACE inhibition	Blood pressure regulation
Soy Peptides	Reduced intestinal absorption/metabolism	Cholesterol management
Melanotan-II	Anti-inflammatory	Reduced risk of atherosclerosis
Glutathione	Antioxidant	Protection against oxidative stress
Thymosin Beta-4	Tissue repair/regeneration	Enhanced recovery post-heart injury
B-type Natriuretic Pp	Blood pressure/Fluid balance regulation	Management of heart failure symptoms

Peptides and Autoimmune Disorders

Autoimmune disorders occur when the body's immune system mistakenly attacks its own cells and tissues. Instead of defending against harmful invaders such as bacteria and viruses, the immune system targets healthy body parts, leading to inflammation, pain, and tissue damage. Examples of autoimmune diseases include rheumatoid arthritis, lupus, multiple sclerosis, type 1 diabetes, and inflammatory bowel diseases like Crohn's disease. In recent years, research has shown that peptides could hold promise in treating autoimmune disorders by modulating the immune response and reducing inflammation.

1. **Thymosin Alpha-1**: Thymosin alpha-1 (Tα1) is a peptide derived from the thymus gland. Known for its ability to boost immune function, Tα1 enhances T-cell activity, which plays a crucial role in adaptive immunity. Studies have shown that Tα1 can modulate the immune system by increasing various cytokines that regulate inflammation and immune responses. Its immunomodulatory properties make it an appealing candidate for treating autoimmune conditions such as lupus and multiple sclerosis.

2. **BPC-157**: Body Protection Compound 157 (BPC-157) is a synthetic peptide composed of 15 amino acids. Research indicates that BPC-157 has significant healing properties and anti-inflammatory effects. It has shown promise in treating inflammatory bowel diseases by promoting intestinal health and reducing gut inflammation. The peptide works by influencing growth factors involved in cell repair and regeneration.

3. **LL-37**: LL-37 is an antimicrobial peptide with broad-spectrum antibacterial activity. Apart from its role in fighting infections, LL-37 also modulates the immune response by regulating cytokines and chemokines—molecules pivotal to cell signaling in immune reactions. Given its dual role in fighting pathogens and regulating immunity, LL-37 shows potential in managing autoimmune conditions characterized by aberrant inflammation.

Mechanisms of Action

Autoimmune conditions are complex, involving multiple factors like genetics, environmental triggers, and immune dysregulation. Peptides offer multidimensional approaches to tackle these diseases. Below are some key mechanisms through which peptides can influence autoimmune disorders:

1. **Immune Modulation:** Peptides like Tα1 can rebalance the immune system by enhancing regulatory T-cells while suppressing autoreactive T-cells.
2. **Reduction of Inflammation:** Peptides such as BPC-157 act on inflammatory pathways to lower pro-inflammatory cytokine levels.
3. **Cell Protection:** Many peptides assist in cell renewal and protection against oxidative stress and cellular damage common in autoimmune disorders.
4. **Tissue Repair:** Peptides encourage tissue regeneration by activating growth factors critical for repairing damaged tissues affected by autoimmune attacks.

PEPTIDE	MECHANISM	Potential Application
Thymosin Alpha-1	Immune modulation	Lupus, Multiple Sclerosis
BPC-157	Healing, Anti-inflammatory	Crohn's Disease
LL-37	Antimicrobial, Immune regulation	Rheumatoid Arthritis

While emerging peptide therapies offer exciting possibilities for managing autoimmune disorders, much work remains to be done to translate these findings into standard treatments fully. Clinical trials are necessary to test efficacy and safety comprehensively. Individual responses may vary based on various factors like disease severity, genetic background, and concurrent therapies.

Neurodegenerative Diseases

Neurodegenerative diseases are characterized by the progressive loss of function and structure of neurons. The quest for effective treatments has led researchers to explore peptides due to their ability to modulate biological processes. One promising area of research is the development of peptide-based drugs that can cross the blood-brain barrier, offering targeted treatment with minimal side effects.

Alzheimer's Disease

Alzheimer's disease is the most common neurodegenerative disorder, causing memory loss and cognitive decline. Researchers have investigated various peptides that could potentially mitigate or reverse these effects. For instance, amyloid-beta peptide accumulation in the brain forms plaques that are a hallmark of Alzheimer's. Scientists are exploring peptides that can inhibit or dissolve these plaques.

1. *Beta-Amyloid Peptides:* These peptides aggregate to form plaques. Inhibiting this aggregation is a significant area of research.
2. *Tau Proteins:* Hyperphosphorylation of tau proteins leads to tangles inside neurons. Modifying peptide interactions here can reduce tangle formation.

Parkinson's Disease

Parkinson's disease involves the degeneration of dopamine-producing neurons in the brain. Peptides have shown promise in protecting these neurons and enhancing their function.

1. *Nurr1 Peptide:* This peptide plays a role in maintaining dopamine levels by promoting the survival of dopamine-producing neurons.
2. *Glucagon-like Peptide-1 (GLP-1):* This peptide has been observed to have neuroprotective effects, reducing inflammation and oxidative stress in neuronal cells.

Amyotrophic Lateral Sclerosis (ALS)

ALS is characterized by the degeneration of motor neurons leading to muscle weakness and atrophy. Peptide-based approaches are being explored to delay disease progression.

1. **Cyclic Peptides:** These are designed to stabilize protein structures, preventing misfolding that contributes to neural degeneration.
2. **SOD1 Peptides:** Mutations in Superoxide Dismutase 1 (SOD1) are linked to ALS. Targeted peptides can help correct these mutations' effects.

Therapeutic Developments

Peptide-based therapies offer several advantages over traditional drug designs, including specificity and fewer side effects. Key developments include:

1. **Peptide Inhibitors:** These prevent harmful protein interactions or aggregations.
2. **Peptidomimetics:** Designed to mimic peptide structures with enhanced stability and efficacy.

DISEASE	PEPTIDE	FUNCTION/EFFECT
Alzheimer's	Beta-Amyloid, Tau	Plaque inhibition, tangle reduction
Parkinson's	Nurr1, GLP-1	Dopamine neuron protection, anti-inflammatory
ALS	Cyclic Peptides, SOD1	Protein stabilization, mutation correction

The ongoing research into peptides opens doors to understanding and potentially treating neurodegenerative diseases more effectively. While much work remains to be done, peptides hold significant promise as part of future therapeutic strategies for enhancing longevity and well-being for those suffering from these debilitating conditions. This simplified overview reflects current advancements and potential directions for peptide-based treatments within neurodegenerative diseases.

Diabetes Management

Diabetes is a chronic condition that affects how the body turns food into energy. Insulin is the primary hormone involved in this process, and its dysfunction plays a central role in diabetes. Since insulin itself is a peptide hormone, it highlights the importance of peptides in diabetes treatment. However, recent advances have uncovered various other peptides that can help manage blood sugar levels, improve insulin sensitivity, and even possibly regenerate beta cells (the cells responsible for producing insulin).

1. **GLP-1 Agonists**: One class of peptides that has garnered significant attention is GLP-1 agonists. GLP-1, or glucagon-like peptide-1, is naturally produced in the gut and enhances insulin secretion post-meal. Synthetic versions of this peptide, known as GLP-1 agonists (e.g., Exendin-4), mimic its natural effects but last longer in the body.

   a. *Improved glycemic control:* Helps maintain stable blood glucose levels.
   b. *Weight loss:* Reduces appetite and delays gastric emptying.
   c. *Cardiovascular benefits:* Lowers the risk of heart disease.

2. **Amylin Analogs**: Amylin is another peptide that works alongside insulin to regulate blood sugar levels. Pramlintide (a synthetic analog of amylin) has been developed to aid people with both Type 1 and Type 2 diabetes.

   a. *Glucose Control:* Smooths out postprandial glucose spikes.
   b. *Weight Management:* Promotes satiety.

3. **DPP-IV Inhibitors**: Dipeptidyl peptidase-IV (DPP-IV) inhibitors work by blocking the enzyme that degrades GLP-1. By doing so, they increase the levels and activity of endogenous GLP-1.

   a. *Enhanced Insulin Response:* Increases insulin secretion.
   b. *Decreased Glucagon Levels:* Lowers blood sugar production by inhibiting glucagon.

Emerging research suggests certain peptides may foster beta-cell regeneration or protect existing beta cells from damage. For instance, C-peptide is being investigated for its potential to repair damaged beta cells and reduce complications related to diabetes like neuropathy.

PEPTIDE	FUNCTION/EFFECT	BENEFITS
Insulin	Regulates blood glucose	Essential for Type 1; necessary for advanced Type 2
GLP-1 Agonists	Enhances insulin secretion	Glycemic control, weight loss, cardiovascular health
Amylin Analogs	Modulates postprandial glucose levels	Reduced glucose spikes, weight management
DPP-IV Inhibitors	Prolongs action of endogenous GLP-1	Enhanced insulin response, lower glucagon levels
C-Peptide	Potential beta-cell regeneration/protection	May aid in reducing diabetic complications	

CHAPTER 3

PEPTIDES AND MENTAL HEALTH

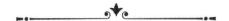

Peptides have a big impact on mental health. They help with thinking, reducing stress and anxiety, improving mood, and getting better sleep. They also support addiction recovery. Knowing how peptides work in these areas can lead to new treatments for better mental health. Peptides are important because they can make our brains work better, make us feel happier, and help us relax more easily. Better understanding of peptides can help in finding new ways to treat different mental health issues.

Enhancing Cognitive Function

One area where peptides have shown promise is in enhancing cognitive function. This is particularly important as we age, since cognitive decline is a common concern. Certain peptides can improve memory, attention, and overall brain performance. For instance, Dihexa is a peptide known for its cognitive-enhancing properties. Research has shown that Dihexa can help in the repair of neural connections, making it useful for conditions like Alzheimer's disease. This peptide enhances synaptogenesis, which is the formation of synapses between neurons in the nervous system. Synapses are vital for communication within the brain, so their formation and maintenance are crucial for learning and memory.

Another peptide worth mentioning is Cerebrolysin. This peptide has been used to treat various neurodegenerative conditions. It helps by promoting the survival of neurons and encourages the growth of new nerve cells and synapses. Studies have indicated that patients using Cerebrolysin showed improvements in cognitive functions such as better memory retention and increased mental clarity.

PEPTIDE	Primary Benefit	Conditions Targeted

Dihexa	Repairing neural connections	Alzheimer's disease
Cerebrolysin	Promoting neuron survival	Neurodegenerative conditions
Semax	Enhancing learning ability	Cognitive impairment

Semax is another peptide known for its nootropic effects, meaning it enhances learning and memory while also having neuroprotective properties. It has been used in Russia to treat patients with cognitive impairments, stroke recovery cases, and even for boosting performance in healthy individuals. Altogether, these peptides present a promising future for addressing cognitive decline and enhancing mental clarity.

Stress and Anxiety Reduction

Stress and anxiety are common problems that many people face today. These issues not only affect mental well-being but can also lead to physical health problems over time. Peptides have shown significant potential in reducing stress and anxiety levels.

One of the well-documented peptides for reducing anxiety is Selank. This peptide modulates the immune system while also producing anxiolytic (anxiety-reducing) effects. Unlike traditional anti-anxiety medications that may cause side effects like drowsiness or addiction, Selank provides relief without these drawbacks.

PT-141, although primarily known for treating sexual dysfunctions like erectile dysfunction and low libido, has also been found to reduce stress levels effectively due to its action on melanocortin receptors which influence mood regulation.

PEPTIDE	Primary Benefit	Secondary Effects
Selank	Reducing anxiety	Immune system modulation
PT-141	Lowering stress levels	Enhanced mood

Another peptide worth noting is DSIP (Delta Sleep-Inducing Peptide). As the name suggests, DSIP helps with sleep regulation which indirectly helps reduce stress levels by improving sleep quality. Poor sleep often exacerbates stress and anxiety; thus improved sleep can lead to overall better mental health. Oxytocin is commonly known as the "love hormone" due to its role in social bonding; however, it also plays a significant role in reducing stress levels. Studies have shown that oxytocin can lower cortisol levels (the stress hormone) in the body, leading to a feeling of calmness and well-being. The adaptability of these peptides provides a wealth of opportunities for developing tailored treatments catered to individual needs.

Mood Improvement

Our mood is influenced by several factors, including neurotransmitter balance, stress levels, and overall brain health. Peptides can positively impact these factors in various ways:

1. **Neurotransmitter Regulation:** Certain peptides help regulate neurotransmitters like serotonin and dopamine, which are critical for mood stabilization. For example:

a. *Selank:* This peptide works by impacting the anxiety-related chemical systems in the brain, leading to reduced anxiety and better mood.

b. *Semax:* Known to enhance cognitive function and has an antidepressant effect by modulating brain-derived neurotrophic factor (BDNF).

2. **Stress Reduction:** Chronic stress can lead to mood disorders such as depression and anxiety. Peptides like:

a. *Thymosin Beta-4:* Help reduce inflammation and promote tissue repair, indirectly reducing the stress on the body.

b. *Corticotropin-Releasing Factor (CRF) Antagonists:* These peptides help manage the body's response to stress by controlling cortisol levels.

3. Enhanced Neuroplasticity: Some peptides promote neuroplasticity, which is the brain's ability to adapt and reorganize itself:

a. *Dihexa:* Has been shown to enhance synaptogenesis (formation of synapses between neurons), aiding cognitive functions that underpin mood regulation.

4. **Balancing Sleep-Wake Cycle:** Quality sleep is integral to mental health and a balanced mood. Improving sleep through peptides helps stabilize moods.

PEPTIDE	FUNCTION	BENEFIT
Selank	Anxiety regulation	Better mood
Semax	Cognitive enhancement & BDNF modulation	Antidepressant effects
Thymosin Beta-4	Reducing inflammation	Lower stress
Corticotropin Releasing Factor Antagonists	Cortisol management	Manage stress
Dihexa	Enhanced neuroplasticity	Improved cognitive functions

Sleep Quality Enhancement

Sleep is fundamental to mental health. Quality sleep allows the body to repair itself and the brain to process information efficiently.

1. **Regulating Sleep Cycles:** Peptides can help regulate sleep-wake cycles:

a. *DSIP (Delta Sleep-Inducing Peptide):* Promotes deep sleep phases necessary for restorative rest.

2. **Enhancing Deep Sleep:** Deep sleep is essential for overall health. Some peptides can enhance sleep depth:

a. *CJC-1295/Ipamorelin Combo:* While primarily known for promoting growth hormone release, these peptides can improve deep sleep cycles.

3. **Hormonal Balance for Better Sleep:** Hormones play a pivotal role in sleep patterns:

a. *Melatonin-related Peptides:* Help regulate circadian rhythms, aiding in more consistent sleep patterns.

4. **Reducing Insomnia Factors:** Many experience poor sleep due to insomnia or fragmented sleep:

a. *GHRH (Growth Hormone-Releasing Hormone):* Can aid in promoting better-quality sleep.

PEPTIDE	FUNCTION	BENEFIT
DSIP	Promotes deep sleep phases	Restorative rest
CJC-1295/Ipamorelin	Growth hormone release	Improved deep sleep cycles
Melatonin-related Peptides	Regulate circadian rhythms	Consistent sleep patterns
GHRH	Promotes better-quality sleep	Reduced insomnia

Addiction and Recovery Support

Traditionally, recovery support has focused on behavioral therapy, counseling, and medications to manage withdrawal symptoms and prevent relapse. However, recent studies have begun exploring the potential role of peptides in addiction treatment and recovery support.

One of the most studied peptides in addiction treatment is Oxytocin. Oxytocin, often called the *"love hormone,"* is known for its role in social bonding, stress reduction, and emotional regulation. Research has shown that oxytocin can decrease cravings and withdrawal symptoms in individuals battling addictions to substances like alcohol, opioids, and even nicotine. The calming effect of oxytocin can help reduce anxiety and stress levels during detoxification, making the initial stages of recovery more manageable.

Another peptide receiving attention is Glutathione. This peptide acts as a powerful antioxidant and detoxifier in the body. Chronic substance abuse often leads to oxidative stress and significant damage to cells. By supplementing with Glutathione, individuals may find support in reversing some damage caused by long-term substance abuse. Improved cellular health alongside traditional recovery methods can enhance overall well-being during recovery.

Moreover, beta-Endorphin is another peptide showing promise in addiction treatment. Beta-Endorphins are natural painkillers produced by the pituitary gland in response to stress or pain. These peptides act on opioid receptors in the brain similar to drugs like morphine but without addictive properties. Increasing levels of beta-Endorphin can naturally alleviate some craving sensations while promoting feelings of well-being.

Corticotropin-Releasing Factor (CRF) is a peptide involved in stress responses. High levels of CRF are often found in people going through withdrawal, leading to heightened anxiety and relapse risk. Blocking CRF receptors has been found to reduce withdrawal symptoms significantly, aiding those attempting long-term sobriety.

In addition to specific peptides, there's ongoing research into combining peptides with more conventional treatment methods for synergetic effects. For example:

TREATMENT COMBINATION	POTENTIAL BENEFIT
Oxytocin + Counseling	Enhanced emotional stability
Glutathione + Detox	Reduced cellular damage from oxidative stress
Beta-Endorphin + CRF Blockers	Natural pain relief with reduced anxiety

It's important to note that while peptide therapy for addiction is promising, it remains an emerging field requiring further clinical trials for robust validation. However, incorporating peptides into established treatment protocols could significantly enhance recovery outcomes.

CHAPTER 4

WOMEN'S AND MEN'S HEALTH

In particular, peptides are invaluable in promoting well-being as we age by aiding in hormonal balance, improving reproductive health, and enhancing sexual function. For women, peptides are essential in managing the complex hormonal changes that occur during menopause. They help regulate hormones like estrogen and progesterone, mitigating symptoms such as hot flashes, night sweats, and mood swings. Similarly, for men, peptides assist in addressing the issues associated with andropause, such as decreased testosterone levels, muscle mass loss, and reduced energy levels.

Both sexes can benefit from peptides that enhance sexual health by improving blood flow, libido, and overall performance. Additionally, peptides are significant in fertility support for both men and women; they help promote healthy ovarian function and sperm quality. This holistic approach ensures that peptides provide a broad spectrum of benefits for maintaining health across different stages of life.

Peptides in Reproductive Health

Peptides have emerged as a promising tool in the field of reproductive health for both men and women. These small proteins play a crucial role in various physiological processes and can be utilized to address specific health issues related to reproduction.

Women's Reproductive Health

In women's reproductive health, peptides have shown potential in addressing conditions such as Polycystic Ovary Syndrome (PCOS) and infertility. For example, Kisspeptin is a peptide that has been found to stimulate the release of gonadotropin-releasing hormone (GnRH), which is essential for the secretion of luteinizing hormone (LH) and follicle-stimulating hormone (FSH). These hormones are critical for ovulation and fertility.

Another peptide, Gonadotropin-Releasing Hormone Agonists (GnRHa), is used to treat endometriosis and fibroids by regulating menstrual cycles and reducing estrogen production. By intervening in these hormone pathways, peptides can help manage symptoms and improve the quality of life for women suffering from these conditions.

PEPTIDE	USE CASE	FUNCTION
Kisspeptin	Infertility	Stimulates GnRH release for ovulation
GnRH Agonists (GnRHa)	Endometriosis, PCOS, Fibroids	Regulates menstrual cycles, reduces estrogen

Men's Reproductive Health

For men, peptides also offer valuable benefits in addressing issues such as low testosterone levels, erectile dysfunction, and infertility. Human Chorionic Gonadotropin (HCG) acts similarly to LH in stimulating testosterone production in the testes. This can be particularly beneficial for men with hypogonadism or those undergoing testosterone replacement therapy.

Another notable peptide, BPC-157, aids in healing by promoting angiogenesis and protecting tissues. It has also shown effectiveness in improving blood flow and healing damaged erectile tissues.

PEPTIDE	USE CASE	FUNCTION
Human Chorionic Gonadotropin (HCG)	Low testosterone	Stimulates testosterone production
BPC-157	Erectile dysfunction	Promotes tissue healing

Addressing Menopause and Andropause

Menopause and Andropause mark significant shifts in hormonal balance that come with aging. These life stages can lead to various symptoms that impact overall health and well-being.

Menopause usually occurs between ages 45-55 when a woman's ovaries stop producing eggs, leading to decreased levels of estrogen and progesterone. This hormonal change results in symptoms such as hot flashes, mood swings, sleep disorders, and vaginal dryness. Peptides like Melanotan II can help alleviate some menopause-related symptoms by reducing hot flashes due to its thermoregulatory properties. Additionally, Thymosin Beta-4 has shown promise in supporting collagen production which aids skin elasticity that often diminishes during menopause.

PEPTIDE	USE CASE	FUNCTION
Melanotan II	Hot flashes	Reduces heat sensitivity
Thymosin Beta-4	Skin elasticity	Supports collagen production

Andropause refers to the gradual decline of testosterone levels in men typically around their 40s or 50s. It manifests through symptoms like fatigue, depression, reduced libido, and muscle mass loss. Peptides such as Growth Hormone-

Releasing Hormone (GHRH) analogs can help combat some effects of Andropause by stimulating the growth hormone axis to promote muscle health, decrease fat mass while increasing energy levels overall.

PEPTIDE	USE CASE	FUNCTION
GHRH Analogs	Muscle health, Energy	Stimulates growth hormone production

Hormonal Regulation

Hormonal regulation is a critical aspect of both women's and men's health. Hormones serve as the body's chemical messengers, influencing various functions, ranging from mood and energy levels to reproductive health. Understanding hormonal balance is key to enhancing well-being and longevity.

In women, hormones such as estrogen, progesterone, and testosterone play significant roles. Estrogen is primarily responsible for sexual development and reproductive health. Its levels fluctuate throughout a woman's menstrual cycle, affecting mood, energy levels, and overall well-being. Progesterone prepares the uterus for pregnancy after ovulation, maintaining the uterine lining for a fertilized egg. An imbalance in these hormones can lead to issues such as premenstrual syndrome (PMS), polycystic ovary syndrome (PCOS), and menopause symptoms like hot flashes and night sweats. Hormonal therapies, dietary changes, and lifestyle adjustments can help manage these imbalances.

In men, testosterone is the primary hormone influencing sexual development, muscle mass, bone density, and mood. Testosterone levels naturally decline with age, which can affect libido, energy levels, and overall vitality. Low testosterone (low-T) can lead to conditions such as hypogonadism, characterized by low energy, depression, reduced muscle mass, and infertility. Treatments such as testosterone replacement therapy (TRT), exercise, nutrition optimization, and lifestyle changes can help manage low-T symptoms.

COMPARISON TABLE OF KEY HORMONES			
	PRIMARY HORMONES	FUNCTIONS	COMMON IMBALANCES
Women	Estrogen; Progesterone	Sexual development; Reproductive health; Mood regulation	PMS; PCOS; Menopause
Men	Testosterone	Sexual development; Maintaining muscle mass; Bone density	Low libido; Low energy; Depression

Sexual Health Enhancement

Sexual health is a crucial component of overall well-being for both men and women. It encompasses not only physical aspects but also emotional and psychological factors. Women's sexual health involves a complex interplay of hormonal balance, psychological well-being, and relational factors. Key areas of concern include libido, sexual arousal disorders, pain during intercourse (dyspareunia), and vaginismus (involuntary tightening of the vaginal muscles).

Hormones such as estrogen play a vital role in maintaining vaginal lubrication and elasticity which affects sexual comfort. Testosterone also contributes to libido in women. Interventions may include hormone replacement therapy (HRT), pelvic floor exercises, counseling or therapy for underlying psychological issues.

For men, common concerns include erectile dysfunction (ED), premature ejaculation (PE), low libido, and performance anxiety. Testosterone again plays a vital role in sexual health by affecting libido and erectile function. Erectile dysfunction may be addressed through medications such as phosphodiesterase inhibitors (Viagra or Cialis), lifestyle changes (exercise to improve cardiovascular health), or addressing underlying conditions like diabetes or hypertension which affect blood flow. Psychological support can also be beneficial in managing performance anxiety or relationship issues contributing to sexual problems.

COMPARISON STRATEGIES FOR ENHANCEMENT		
	COMMON ISSUES	**ENHANCEMENTS**
Women	Libido reduction; Sexual arousal disorders; Dyspareunia	Hormone replacement therapy; Pelvic floor exercises; Counseling/therapy
Men	Erectile dysfunction; Premature ejaculation; Low libido	Phosphodiesterase inhibitors (e.g., Viagra, Cialis); Psychological support; Targeting underlying conditions

Fertility Support

In the quest for enhanced fertility, both women and men benefit from a deeper understanding of the role that peptides play in reproductive health. Certain peptides have exhibited remarkable abilities to support and improve fertility through various mechanisms that address hormonal imbalances and optimize reproductive functions.

For women, peptides like Kisspeptin are vital in regulating the menstrual cycle and ovulation. Kisspeptin stimulates the release of Gonadotropin-Releasing Hormone (GnRH) from the hypothalamus, which in turn triggers the release of Follicle-Stimulating Hormone (FSH) and Luteinizing Hormone (LH) from the pituitary gland. These hormones are crucial for the development and release of eggs from the ovaries. By promoting regular menstrual cycles and healthy ovulation, Kisspeptin can significantly enhance female fertility.

Men also stand to gain substantially from peptide therapy aimed at boosting fertility. Human Chorionic Gonadotropin (hCG) is one such peptide that mimics Luteinizing Hormone (LH) in men. LH is necessary for stimulating testosterone production in the testes. Adequate levels of testosterone not only support overall male health but also improve sperm production and motility, thereby enhancing male fertility.

Both men and women can benefit from optimized nutritional status when trying to conceive. The inclusion of antioxidant-rich foods can protect reproductive cells from oxidative stress, which can impair fertility. For instance, vitamins C and E, along with minerals like zinc and selenium, play a significant role in maintaining healthy eggs and sperm.

Peptide	Role in Women	Role in Men
Kisspeptin	Regulates menstrual cycles	-
Human Chorionic Gonadotropin (hCG)	-	Stimulates testosterone production
Gonadotropin-Releasing Hormone (GnRH)	Triggers FSH & LH release	Triggers FSH & LH release

CHAPTER 5

AN INTRODUCTION TO CELLULAR SENESCENCE

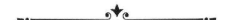

Cellular senescence is a natural process where cells stop dividing and enter a state of permanent growth arrest without dying. This is important in our understanding of aging and age-related diseases, as well as in the field of longevity. Cells divide and grow throughout our lives, but they can't do so indefinitely. At some point, they reach their limit, known as the Hayflick limit, named after Dr. Leonard Hayflick who discovered this mechanism in the 1960s. Usually, this limit is about 40 to 60 divisions for a human cell before it enters senescence.

Senescence can be triggered by several factors. One major cause is telomere shortening. Telomeres are protective caps at the end of our chromosomes that get shorter each time a cell divides. When they become too short, the cell recognizes this as damage and stops dividing to prevent potential mutations that can lead to cancer.

Another trigger for cellular senescence is DNA damage caused by external factors like UV radiation or internal stressors like reactive oxygen species (ROS). The cell activates its damage response pathways to halt division and repair itself. If the damage is irreparable, the cell may enter senescence to avoid passing on faulty DNA.

While cellular senescence serves as an important anti-cancer mechanism by stopping damaged cells from proliferating uncontrollably, it isn't without its downsides. Accumulated senescent cells release inflammatory signals and other molecules that can harm neighboring cells, contributing to aging-related diseases such as arthritis, cardiovascular disease, and even neurodegenerative disorders like Alzheimer's disease.

Researchers have found ways senescent cells achieve such impacts through something called the Senescence-Associated Secretory Phenotype (SASP). SASP involves the release of pro-inflammatory cytokines, chemokines, growth factors, and proteases that collectively create a harmful environment within tissues.

Interestingly, not all senescent cells are harmful; some play critical roles in wound healing and development by secreting factors that help these processes. However, problems arise when too many senescent cells accumulate over time and are not cleared away properly by the immune system.

To combat these negative effects, scientists are exploring several approaches. One promising area of research lies in drugs called senolytics. Senolytics selectively eliminate senescent cells while leaving healthy cells unharmed. Studies in mice have shown that clearing these cells can reduce signs of aging and extend lifespan. Another strategy focuses on modulating SASP with compounds known as SASP inhibitors or modulators which aim to curb the harmful secretions from senescent cells without killing them outright.

Understanding how cellular senescence works gives us valuable insights into aging and holds promise for developing interventions that enhance longevity and healthspan—that portion of life spent free from chronic disease and disability.

The Intelligence of the Cell

Cells, the fundamental units of life, exhibit a remarkable level of intelligence. They respond to their environment, repair damage, communicate with each other, and manage energy production efficiently. A particularly fascinating aspect of cellular behavior is how they deal with stress and damage—this is where cellular senescence comes in.

Cell Senescence

Cellular senescence is a response to various forms of cellular stress such as DNA damage, oxidative stress, or oncogene activation. When cells encounter such stressors, they can either repair the damage or induce controlled death (apoptosis). However, sometimes cells opt for a third option—senescence. In this state, cells cease to proliferate to prevent potential tumor development caused by damaged DNA but remain metabolically active.

Senescent cells release chemical signals known as the senescence-associated secretory phenotype (SASP). This secretion can lead to inflammation and impact neighboring cells negatively if senescent cells accumulate over time. While initially beneficial—playing roles in wound healing and reducing cancer risks—persistent senescent cells contribute to aging and age-related diseases like arthritis and cardiovascular diseases.

Hormesis

Hormesis is another fascinating concept related to cellular response that underscores the adaptability and intelligence of our cells. Hormesis refers to the idea that low doses of a harmful substance or mild stress stimulate adaptive beneficial effects on the cell or organism. Essentially, what doesn't kill them makes them stronger.

For example, mild oxidative stress can trigger an adaptive response that increases the overall resistance of cells to subsequent more severe stress. It essentially enhances their ability to cope with future challenges. Exercise is a practical example of hormesis at work; regular physical activity induces mild oxidative stress but leads over time to improved endurance and muscle strength through adaptive responses.

Connecting Cellular Senescence and Hormesis

Understanding both cellular senescence and hormesis helps us appreciate the delicate balance within our bodies' cellular environment. When this balance tips too far towards persistent senescence without adequate removal mechanisms like immune clearance or dilution by tissue renewal, chronic inflammation ensues—a contributing factor in aging processes.

Conversely, promoting hormetic processes via lifestyle changes—regular exercise, balanced diet rich in antioxidants—could enhance our body's resilience against harmful stressors while mitigating premature cellular aging effects.

Delaying Senescence and Restoring Cellular Efficiency

Cellular senescence occurs when cells stop dividing but do not die. These cells accumulate in tissues, releasing various chemicals that can cause inflammation and tissue damage, contributing to aging and a variety of diseases such as cancer, osteoarthritis, and atherosclerosis. There are multiple strategies to delay senescence and enhance cellular efficiency:

1. **Lifestyle Changes:** Regular physical activity, a balanced diet rich in antioxidants, and proper hydration can mitigate the impact of cellular aging.
2. **Caloric Restriction:** Limiting calorie intake without malnutrition has shown to delay the aging process in various organisms.
3. **Pharmacological Approaches:** Drugs like senolytics can selectively eliminate senescent cells to reduce their harmful effects.

Emerging therapies seek to restore cellular efficiency by rejuvenating these aged cells or replacing them with fresh, functional ones. One promising avenue involves harnessing growth hormones to improve cellular function.

Harnessing Growth Hormone to Improve Cellular Efficiency

Growth hormone (GH) is crucial for growth during childhood and continues to influence health throughout life. Recent studies highlight its role in maintaining tissue and organ function by promoting cell growth, regeneration, and repair. Growth hormone is produced by the pituitary gland at the base of the brain. It stimulates growth, cell reproduction, and regeneration in humans. This hormone acts on various tissues including bones and muscles:

1. **Stimulating Protein Synthesis:** GH promotes the creation of proteins which are essential for repairing tissues.
2. **Boosting Metabolism:** It increases the rate at which fats are broken down to use as energy.
3. **Enhancing Cell Growth:** GH stimulates the growth of bones and muscles by increasing the number of new cells.

Over time, natural production of GH declines which coincides with symptoms of aging such as muscle loss, reduced bone density, and decreased overall vitality.

GHRH/GHRP: How You Can Restore Cell Efficiency

Growth Hormone-Releasing Hormone (GHRH) and Growth Hormone-Releasing Peptides (GHRP) are compounds that encourage your body to release more GH naturally:

1. **Growth Hormone-Releasing Hormone (GHRH):** GHRH stimulates the pituitary gland directly to produce more GH. It enhances sleep quality which is crucial since most GH release occurs during deep sleep.

2. **Growth Hormone-Releasing Peptides (GHRP):** GHRPs act on ghrelin receptors which help release stored GH. They have an additional role in stimulating appetite which can aid those suffering from malnutrition or muscle wasting conditions.

By restoring GH levels through these methods, one can potentially rejuvenate cells leading to improved repair mechanisms, better muscle mass maintenance, enhanced energy levels, and overall improved quality of life.

Current research indicates that using GHRH/GHRP not only boosts GH levels but also improves mitochondrial function within cells—the powerhouse generating energy—thereby enhancing cell efficiency overall.

Strengthening the Immune System Against Viruses, Bacteria, and Other Pathogens

The immune system is made up of various cells and proteins that work together to protect the body. It can be divided into two main parts: the innate immune system and the adaptive immune system. The innate immune system is our first line of defense and responds quickly to invaders. It includes physical barriers like the skin and mucous membranes, as well as immune cells that attack invaders on sight. The adaptive immune system, on the other hand, takes longer to respond but provides a stronger and more specific defense against pathogens by remembering previous infections. To keep our immune system functioning optimally, we can take several practical steps:

1. **Healthy Diet:** A diet rich in fruits, vegetables, whole grains, lean proteins, and healthy fats provides essential nutrients that support immune function. Vitamins such as C and D, minerals like zinc, and antioxidants are particularly important for maintaining a strong immune response. Citrus fruits, berries, nuts, seeds, fish, eggs, and green leafy vegetables are excellent choices.

2. **Regular Exercise:** Physical activity increases blood circulation, which helps immune cells move through the body more efficiently. Regular exercise also reduces inflammation and promotes good cardiovascular health—both of which are key for a robust immune system. Aim for at least 30 minutes of moderate exercise most days of the week.

3. **Adequate Sleep:** Quality sleep is vital for immune function. During sleep, the body produces cytokines—proteins that help fight infection and inflammation. Lack of sleep can reduce the production of these protective proteins and weaken the body's ability to fight off illness. Adults should aim for 7-9 hours of uninterrupted sleep per night.

4. **Stress Management:** Chronic stress can suppress the immune response by releasing cortisol—a hormone that reduces inflammation but also lowers immunity with prolonged exposure. Mindfulness techniques such as meditation, deep breathing exercises, yoga, or even hobbies can help manage stress levels effectively.

5. **Hydration:** Staying well-hydrated helps all bodily functions work properly—including the immune system. Water aids in producing lymph, which carries white blood cells throughout your body to fight infection.

6. **Hygiene Practices:** Simple practices like frequent handwashing with soap and water for at least 20 seconds can significantly reduce your risk of infection by removing pathogens before they enter your body.

7. **Vaccinations:** Vaccines are one of the most effective ways to boost your immune system by preparing it to recognize and combat specific pathogens without causing disease itself.

8. **Avoiding Harmful Behaviors:** Smoking weakens the respiratory tract's barrier function against infections and impairs overall immunity. Excessive alcohol consumption can have a similarly detrimental effect by reducing white blood cell counts.

9. **Sunlight Exposure:** Moderate exposure to sunlight boosts vitamin D levels naturally—a nutrient crucial for a healthy immune response.

By incorporating these practices into daily life, you can significantly enhance your body's ability to fend off infections from viruses, bacteria, and other pathogens effectively.

Peptides Targeting GH and IGF Pathways to Reenter the Cell Cycle

Growth hormone (GH) and insulin-like growth factor (IGF) pathways play distinct yet interconnected roles in cellular functions, particularly concerning growth, development, and metabolic processes. Researchers and clinicians have been exploring these pathways for their potential to reinvigorate the cell cycle, offering promising strategies for enhancing longevity, vitality, and overall well-being.

1. **GH Pathway and GHRH Pleiotropic Effects**: Growth Hormone-Releasing Hormone (GHRH) has a broad range of effects on the body, extending far beyond its primary role in stimulating the release of Growth Hormone (GH) from the pituitary gland. These pleiotropic effects involve a multitude of physiological processes, including tissue repair, muscle growth, and metabolism. Through these pathways, GHRH not only influences GH secretion but also contributes to cognitive functions and immune modulation.

2. **MOD GRF (1-29)**: Modified Growth Releasing Factor 1-29, also known as MOD GRF (1-29), is a synthetic peptide analogous to GHRH. It precisely targets receptors in the anterior pituitary gland to enhance GH release. The modification at the 29th amino acid enhances its stability and effectiveness, making it an optimal choice for clinical applications aimed at stimulating GH production.

3. **CJC 1295**: CJC 1295 is a long-acting version of GHRH that includes a drug affinity complex (DAC) component. This modification dramatically boosts its half-life, allowing it to sustain elevated levels of GH over time. CJC 1295 interacts directly with receptors in the pituitary gland to promote GH secretion consistently and effectively.

4. **Tesamorelin**: Tesamorelin is another synthetic analog of GHRH. Its primary use is for reducing visceral fat in HIV-infected patients suffering from lipodystrophy. Tesamorelin stimulates the natural production of human growth hormone, which adequately addresses issues related to fat metabolism and distribution patterns commonly seen in such patients.

5. **GHRP: Ghrelin-like Analogs** Growth Hormone-Releasing Peptides (GHRPs) serve as key components in targeting both GH and Insulin-Like Growth Factor (IGF) pathways:

   a. *Ipamorelin:* Known for its minimal side effects while effectively promoting GH release, Ipamorelin mimics ghrelin without significantly affecting appetite.
   b. *GHRP-6:* Notably effective in increasing food intake alongside GH secretion due to its strong mimicking of ghrelin.
   c. *GHRP-2:* Potent enhancer of GH levels with moderate impact on appetite stimulation compared to GHRP-6.

6. **MK677 (Ibutamoren Mesylate)**: MK677 is an oral secretagogue that mimics ghrelin's action on the ghrelin receptor, thus encouraging GH release without affecting cortisol levels adversely. This compound has been shown effective in boosting lean body mass, enhancing sleep quality, and improving bone density.

7. **Epithalon (Epithalon Acetate Tetra-Peptide)**: Epithalon offers unique benefits affecting the cell cycle through telomerase activation. By prolonging telomere length within chromosomes, Epithalon supports cellular health and combats aging-related cell cycle deficits. Although not a direct player in the GH pathway, it complements other peptides by fostering better cellular environments overall.

Cellular Repair: Helping Cells Recover

The human body is a remarkable system, equipped with the ability to repair and regenerate tissues. At the core of these capabilities are specific compounds known as peptides. In this section, we will focus on four key peptides—BPC 157, GHK-Cu, DSIP, and TB4—and explore their roles in cellular repair and recovery.

1. **BPC 157 (Body Protection Compound 157):** BPC 157 is a synthetic peptide derived from a protein found in the stomach. It has garnered attention for its regenerative properties. BPC 157 boosts the body's healing processes by promoting blood vessel growth (angiogenesis), which supplies more oxygen and nutrients to damaged areas. This helps speed up recovery from injuries like tendon tears, muscle strains, and even ligament damage. Additionally, it exhibits protective effects on the digestive system, aiding in the healing of gastric ulcers and inflammatory bowel disease.

2. **GHK-Cu (Copper Tripeptide GHK-Cu):** GHK-Cu is a naturally occurring copper peptide found in human plasma. It plays a pivotal role in wound healing and skin regeneration. This peptide helps skin cells produce more collagen, which is essential for skin elasticity and strength. Collagen production decreases with age, leading to wrinkles; GHK-Cu can help by revitalizing aging skin cells. Beyond cosmetic benefits, it also aids in tissue repair by reducing inflammation and facilitating the removal of damaged tissue.

3. **DSIP (Delta Sleep-Inducing Peptide):** DSIP is another intriguing peptide due to its sleep-promoting properties. But its benefits extend beyond helping us get restful sleep. By improving deep sleep quality, DSIP enhances the body's natural ability to repair tissues overnight. Sleep stages such as REM and deep sleep are crucial for cellular repair mechanisms. Using DSIP can optimize these stages, thereby accelerating recovery from wear and tear faced during daily activities or physical exercise.

4. **TB4 (Thymosin Beta 4):** Thymosin Beta 4 is an influential peptide that assists in various regeneration processes. TB4 promotes cell migration by creating new pathways for them to reach damaged tissues quickly. This feature proves particularly effective in healing injuries where speedy cell movement is vital—for instance, after surgeries or accidents requiring rapid tissue regeneration. Furthermore, TB4 has anti-inflammatory benefits that help reduce swelling and promote faster recovery.

Cellular Enhancement and Immune Modulation

Cellular enhancement and immune modulation promise to revolutionize how we approach health by targeting the root causes of disease and aging at the cellular level. Three notable peptides that have garnered significant attention in this realm are Thymosin Alpha 1 (TA1), Thymosin Beta 4 (TB4), Melanotan I, and Melanotan II. Each offers unique benefits that contribute to optimized health and immune function.

1. **TA1 (Thymosin Alpha 1):** TA1 is a peptide that has shown great promise in modulating the immune system. It boosts the body's natural defense mechanisms, making it more effective at combating infections and diseases. TA1 works by stimulating the production of T-cells, which are essential for identifying and attacking pathogens. This peptide is especially beneficial for individuals with weakened immune systems, including those undergoing chemotherapy or suffering from chronic illnesses.

Additionally, TA1 has anti-inflammatory properties, which help reduce inflammation throughout the body. Chronic inflammation is linked to numerous health issues, including autoimmune diseases and various forms of cancer. By reducing inflammation, TA1 not only enhances immune function but also promotes overall cellular health.

2. TB4 (Thymosin Beta 4): TB4 is another powerful peptide known for its regenerative properties. This peptide is abundant in tissues that undergo rapid healing, such as skin and muscle. TB4 plays a pivotal role in wound healing and tissue repair by promoting cell migration and new blood vessel formation. Furthermore, TB4 has anti-inflammatory effects similar to those of TA1. It helps reduce chronic inflammation, thereby protecting cells from long-term damage. By accelerating tissue repair and reducing inflammation, TB4 aids in maintaining the integrity of cells and supporting overall health.

TB4 also assists in heart health by preventing scar tissue formation following heart attacks. This ability to modulate the heart's response to injury makes TB4 an exciting area of research for cardiovascular health.

3. Melanotan I and II: Melanotan I and II are peptides primarily known for their ability to stimulate melanin production, which results in a tan-like appearance to the skin without sun exposure. However, their benefits extend far beyond cosmetic effects. Melanotan peptides have been found to possess immune-modulating properties as well. By enhancing melanin production, they provide a degree of protection against UV radiation, reducing the risk of skin cancer—thereby indirectly supporting cellular health.

Moreover, Melanotan II has shown promise in weight management by suppressing appetite. Weight control is crucial for overall health as obesity is linked to various diseases such as diabetes, cardiovascular disease, and certain cancers.

CHAPTER 6

LIFESTYLE AND LONG-TERM WELLNESS

⸱—————✦————⸱

One of the significant ways peptides contribute to wellness is by promoting cellular repair and regeneration. They help improve the communication between cells, which in turn ensures that the body functions more efficiently. For instance, certain peptides stimulate collagen production, leading to healthier skin and better wound healing. Moreover, peptides like GHRH (Growth Hormone-Releasing Hormone) and GHRP (Growth Hormone-Releasing Peptides) activate the release of growth hormone from the pituitary gland. This hormone is vital for cell regeneration, muscle growth, and fat metabolism. By optimizing these processes, peptides can aid in muscle recovery post-exercise, support fat loss, and help maintain a healthy body composition.

Peptides also influence immune function, making them essential in preparing the body to fight infections and other threats more effectively. By enhancing the immune response, peptides ensure that the body's defense mechanisms are robust enough to combat viruses, bacteria, and even cancer cells. Peptides are indispensable for maintaining lifestyle and long-term wellness through their roles in cellular communication, tissue repair, hormone regulation, and immune function.

Daily Practices for Peptide Users

Adopting daily practices that complement peptide usage can significantly enhance overall wellness and longevity. Here are some effective daily habits:

1. Drinking sufficient water is crucial. Aim for at least 8 glasses of water a day to keep your body hydrated and functioning optimally. Proper hydration can aid in the absorption and effectiveness of peptides.
2. Consuming a diet rich in vitamins, minerals, proteins, and good fats supports body functions and peptide effectiveness. Include plenty of fruits, vegetables, lean proteins, whole grains, and healthy fats in your meals.
3. Engaging in at least 30 minutes of moderate exercise most days helps maintain muscle mass, flexibility, cardiovascular health, and mental well-being. Incorporate a mix of cardio, strength training, and flexibility exercises.
4. : Quality sleep is essential for recovery and overall health. Aim for 7-9 hours of uninterrupted sleep per night. Create a sleep-friendly environment by keeping your bedroom dark, quiet, and cool.
5. Chronic stress can negatively impact your health. Practice stress-reducing techniques such as yoga, meditation, deep breathing exercises, or even hobbies that you enjoy.
6. Regular visits to healthcare professionals help monitor your health status and optimize peptide regimen based on personal needs.

Below is a sample schedule for an individual integrating these practices:

TIME	ACTIVITY
6:00 AM	Drink a glass of water
6:30 AM	Morning exercise (e.g., jogging/yoga)
7:30 AM	Healthy breakfast
12:00 PM	Hydration break + light snack
1:00 PM	Balanced lunch
3:00 PM	Afternoon stretch or walk
6:00 PM	Nutritious dinner
8:00 PM	Relaxation (meditation/reading)
10:00 PM	Prepare for bed

Anti-Aging Lifestyle Integration

Integrating anti-aging principles into daily life can further promote long-term wellness alongside peptide use:

1. **Healthy Eating Patterns:**

    a. *Anti-Inflammatory Foods:* These include berries, fatty fish like salmon, nuts like almonds, olive oil, leafy greens like spinach, tomatoes, etc.

    b. *Antioxidant-Rich Foods:* Such as dark chocolate (in moderation), pecans, blueberries, strawberries.

    c. Reduce Processed Foods that contain high sugar levels or unhealthy fats which can accelerate aging.

2. **Intermittent Fasting (IF):** IF patterns like the 16/8 method (16 hours fasting window with an 8-hour eating period) are reported to enhance cellular repair processes and improve metabolism.

3. **Environmental Factors:** Minimize exposure to pollutants by using air purifiers indoors. Apply sunscreen daily to protect skin from UV radiation damage.

4. **Cognitive Activities:** Keep the brain active through reading, puzzles, learning new skills/hobbies to stave off cognitive decline.

5. **Social Connections:** Positive social interactions contribute significantly to mental well-being; make efforts to stay connected with family/friends.

6. **Supplementation:** Consult with healthcare providers about integrating supplements such as Vitamin D3 which supports bone health or Omega-3 fatty acids beneficial for heart health.

By incorporating these lifestyle choices into your daily routine while using peptides, you have a well-rounded approach to enhancing your longevity, vitality, and overall well-being.

Community and Support Networks

Building a strong community and support network is a vital component for long-term wellness. Connections with others provide both emotional and practical support, which can enhance overall health. Research shows that people with robust social connections have lower risks of several health issues, including heart disease, high blood pressure, and depression. The importance of social connections includes:

1. **Emotional Support:** Having someone to talk to about your experiences, fears, and joys reduces stress and promotes mental well-being.

2. **Practical Support:** Friends, family, or community members can assist with daily tasks or medical care when needed.

3. **Encouragement and Motivation:** A supportive network can motivate you to maintain healthy habits such as regular exercise and balanced diet.

Building Your Network

1. **Family:** Start by strengthening ties with family members. Regular family gatherings or shared activities can build stronger bonds.
2. **Friends:** Keep in touch with friends regularly through calls, texts, or social media. Plan regular meetups or activities together.
3. **Community Groups:** Join local clubs or organizations that align with your interests (e.g., book clubs, sports teams, volunteer groups).

Online Communities

1. **Forums and Social Media Groups:** Many online platforms offer communities where you can share experiences and get advice on wellness.
2. **Virtual Meetups:** Use video calls to maintain connections with distant friends or family.

Below is a simple comparison chart showing the benefits of different types of support networks:

Type of Support	Examples	Benefits
Emotional	Family, close friends	Reduced stress, mental well-being
Practical	Neighbors, colleagues	Assistance with tasks, caregiving
Motivational	Fitness groups, mentors	Encouragement for healthy habits

Longevity Strategies

Incorporating longevity strategies into your lifestyle is crucial for prolonging not just lifespan but also health span—the period during which you remain healthy and active. Here are some effective strategies to enhance longevity:

1. **Caloric Restriction:** Scientific studies suggest that reducing caloric intake without malnutrition can prolong lifespan. It's thought to work by reducing metabolic rates and oxidative damage.

2. **High-Nutrient Diets:** Eating nutrient-dense foods provides essential vitamins, minerals, and antioxidants that support cell function and repair. Examples include leafy greens, berries, nuts, seeds, lean proteins, and legumes.

3. **Mind-Body Connection:** Practices like meditation and mindfulness reduce stress, improve mental health, and have been linked to increased telomere length (a biomarker for aging).

4. **Exercise:** Consistent physical activity helps maintain muscle mass, bone density, cardiovascular health, and metabolic function. Aim for a mix of aerobic (e.g., walking, jogging), strength (e.g., weight lifting), and flexibility exercises (e.g., yoga).

5. **Adequate Sleep:** Quality sleep aids in the repair of cells and regulation of hormones such as melatonin which has anti-aging properties.

6. **Stay Hydrated:** Water is essential for most bodily functions including digestion, circulation, temperature regulation, and cellular repair.

7. **Avoiding Harmful Habits:**

   a. *Smoking Cessation:* Reducing or eliminating tobacco use decreases the risk of heart disease and cancer.

b. *Moderate Alcohol Consumption:* Limit alcohol intake as excessive consumption is linked with various chronic conditions.

8. **Mental Stimulation & Social Interaction:** Engage in activities that stimulate your mind such as puzzles, reading, or learning new skills. Maintain a strong social network to protect against mental decline and promote emotional well-being.

Ethical Considerations for Long-Term Use

When utilizing peptides for enhancing longevity and overall wellness, ethical considerations must come to the forefront. Although peptides can offer tremendous benefits, their long-term usage raises several important ethical issues:

1. Informed Consent: Individuals using peptides should be fully informed about the potential benefits, risks, and side effects associated with their long-term use. This information should be provided by healthcare professionals who are well-versed in peptide therapy.
2. Accessibility: The accessibility of peptide therapy can often be restricted due to costs, making it primarily available to those who can afford it. There needs to be an ethical discussion on making such beneficial treatments more equitable and accessible to a broader population.
3. Regulation and Safety: Ensuring that peptide products are safe and effective is crucial. This involves adhering to stringent regulatory standards set by health authorities. Unregulated or poorly monitored usage could lead to misuse or significant health problems.
4. Potential for Abuse: Long-term use of peptides may lead some individuals to misuse them for performance enhancement beyond therapeutic norms, such as in sports. This not only presents health risks but also raises issues around fairness and integrity in competitive environments.
5. Sustainability: The production and demand for peptides must be balanced with sustainable practices to avoid adverse environmental impacts. Ethical sourcing and manufacturing practices should be promoted.
6. Long-term Impact Studies: There is a need for ongoing research into the long-term impacts of peptide use, including potential unknown side effects or cumulative impacts over time. Patients should be made aware of the current limits of scientific understanding regarding long-term use.

It is essential that these ethical considerations are discussed not just among medical professionals but also within broader societal contexts to ensure responsible usage aligned with public health interests.

CONCLUSION

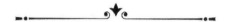

As we close this comprehensive guide on peptide protocols, it's important to reflect on the valuable insights and practical advice shared throughout this book. Peptides have emerged as a powerful tool for enhancing longevity and vitality. Their ability to boost brain health, improve physical performance, strengthen the immune system, and regulate hormonal balance makes them a key player in modern health optimization strategies. By understanding the basics of peptide therapy—from synthesis and administration routes to stability and storage—we can make informed decisions about incorporating these potent biomolecules into our health routines.

One of the book's major highlights is its focus on targeted strategies for different health goals. Whether you're aiming to enhance cognitive function with brain-boosting peptides, support muscle repair and recovery with specific protocols, or boost your immune system against infections, there's a peptide solution tailored to your needs. The detailed protocols provided offer step-by-step guidance and customization options, ensuring that you can craft an effective regimen suited to your individual requirements.

Moreover, integrating peptides with other therapies further amplifies their benefits. Combining them with proper nutrition, lifestyle modifications, pharmaceuticals when necessary, or holistic approaches ensures a comprehensive approach to health. This synergy helps prevent potential interactions and enhances overall well-being.

Tracking and optimizing results play a crucial role in achieving long-term success with peptide use. Utilizing tools like monitoring devices and keeping track of progress helps in interpreting results accurately. Adapting protocols based on these insights ensures that we're always moving towards our health goals effectively.

The future of peptide therapies looks promising with ongoing research frontiers exploring experimental peptides and advanced applications. Understanding genetic considerations and leveraging peptide stacks open new avenues for personalized health interventions. As science progresses, so will our understanding of how best to utilize these peptides for maximum benefit.

Healing properties of peptides cannot be understated—whether it's anti-inflammatory effects aiding in tissue repair and regeneration or neuroprotective properties supporting brain health. Their application in disease management offers hope for those battling chronic conditions like cancer, cardiovascular issues, autoimmune disorders, and neurodegenerative diseases.

Maintaining mental health is another significant area where peptides show immense potential. Enhancing cognitive function, reducing stress and anxiety, improving mood, ensuring quality sleep, and supporting addiction recovery are critical aspects where peptides have shown promising results.

For both men and women, peptides contribute significantly to reproductive health by addressing hormonal imbalances, supporting fertility, and enhancing sexual health. Moreover, understanding cellular senescence—how cells age—and employing strategies to delay it can lead to improved longevity through better cellular efficiency and immune modulation.

Integrating daily practices involving peptides into an anti-aging lifestyle along with community support networks forms a sustainable approach towards long-term wellness. Ethical considerations must always guide this journey as we strive for improved quality of life through the intelligent application of peptide science.

Final advice: Start your peptide journey with a clear goal in mind. Be informed about what peptides suit your needs best; follow evidence-based protocols; monitor your progress diligently; stay updated with ongoing research; always consult healthcare professionals when needed; most importantly—commit to a holistic approach encompassing good nutrition, lifestyle habits alongside your peptide regimen for optimal well-being. Your path to enhanced longevity and vitality is now mapped out—embrace it confidently!

Made in the USA
Las Vegas, NV
07 September 2024

94897977R00063